Normal Blood Test Aren't Good Enough!

"I recommend blood testing with Your Future Health (YFH) to all my patients—including those who are healthy and wish to stay that way."

Tatiana Canning, MD

"Ellie shows that individuals have distinctive Personal Normal scores that are in a much more narrow range than the laboratory's "normals." This tool for early detection of disease is the key to preventing illness."

Dan C. Dantini, MD

"Monitoring blood test results consistently over time can red-flag disease before symptoms occur. This gives patients and their doctors a way to measure lifestyle changes and other interventions early in the course of treatment."

Tamara Sachs, MD

"Ellie's idea of testing your blood to know how to optimize your own nutrition—not anyone else's—just makes sense. And it works."

Vicki Nassif, DDS

"Through Your Future Health and Ellie Cullen I have been able to change my patients' health, as well as my own, in a positive direction. For example, one 32 year-old man's first Omega 3 Profile+ (AA/EPA ratio) test score was high at 50. With the right amount of fish oil, as determined by the test, his next ratio was better at 2.0. His symptoms improved from not feeling good, to feeling noticeably, much better.

Underlying "silent inflammation" is the root cause of all chronic diseases such as Cardiovascular, Osteoarthritis, Osteoporosis, Dementia, Diabetes, Cancer, etc. Specific laboratory tests through Your Future Health and Ellie's guidance can prevent these chronic conditions."

Ashok G. Patel, MD, Family Practice

"Ellie's pioneering work will save your health and your money—it might even save your life!"

Frankie Boyer, Health Writer and Radio Host:
"The Frankie Boyer Show" & "The Woman's Show" on Sirius

"Ellie is the Johnny Appleseed of preventive blood testing."

Oscar Rasmussen, PhD

"For everyone who cares about being healthy, this book is a must read!"

E. Martin Hecklinger, CEO, Sage Systems, Inc.

Normal

Blood Test Scores Aren't Good Enough!

A Layman's Guide to Understanding Preventive Blood Testing

~~~~~~~~~~~~~~~~~

Ellie Cullen, RN

2nd Edition

~~~~~~~~~~~~~~~~~

YFH Press 2002-2004

http://www.yourfuturehealth.com

Library of Congress Cataloging-in-Publication Data
Normal Blood Test Scores Aren't Good Enough! / Cullen, Ellie
p. cm.
Includes index.
ISBN 0-9716283-0-0

ATTENTION: ORGANIZATIONS AND CORPORATIONS

This book is available at special quantity discounts
for bulk purchases. For information, please call or write:

Special Markets Department, YFH Press
P.O. Box 1369, Tavares, FL 32778

Toll free 877-468-6934   **Fax 352-253-0794**

Printed in the United States of America
First Printing February, 2002
Second Printing May, 2003
Third Printing September, 2003
Fourth Printing, Second Edition August, 2004
Cover design and illustrations by Mark Anderson

This book is affectionately dedicated to Emanuel Cheraskin, MD, DMD, an internationally renowned scientist and educator, who passed away on the 3rd of August 2001 in his eighty-fifth year. He was an extraordinary human being with a vibrant one-of-a-kind sense of humor.

Dr. Cheraskin was one of the pioneering advocates of the health benefits of vitamin C. A prolific researcher and writer, his twenty-five books (seventeen of which were textbooks) and over seven hundred published scientific studies in peer review journals regularly broke new ground within nutrition, dental health, chelation therapy, and vitamin/mineral supplementation fields. "Cherrie," as he was known to his close friends, always hoped that his writings would expand the medical community's understanding of health and wellness; and at this, he was extremely successful. Scores of his findings and insights are now a part of the medical status quo.

It would be difficult to overestimate Dr. Cheraskin's inspiring influence on my work over the years. I can only hope that the reader will garner some small portion of the same insight his works provided me in the pages I have written here.

Acknowledgments

I would first like to thank YFH's many clients, who not only encouraged me to develop this book, but some of whom contributed their time, and with only the goal of helping others, allowed intimate and personal details of their lives to be revealed.

My sincere and heartfelt thanks also go to the many doctors and medical practitioners, especially Dr. Oscar Rasmussen, who reviewed this manuscript and offered dozens of useful suggestions.

I especially wish to thank Ann Louise Gittleman, Burton Goldberg and Betty Kamen for their kind and gracious contributions. Betty has been a wonderful mentor. She has continually challenged me to make this book the best that it could be. And of course the talented David Hennessy, who edited my thoughts with polish and precision.

An emotional thank you to my two children, Maureen and Brian, and their spouses, Remo and Kristen, for their tireless support and help with the manuscript. An extra hug to Brian, who left P&G to help expand our company to meet the needs of our rapid growth. And most of all, deep thanks and appreciation to my husband, Terry Cullen, soul mate, partner, and wind beneath my sails.

Foreword
Ann Louise Gittleman PhD, CNS

In over twenty years of counseling and researching, I've come to one conclusion. We are not created equal... biochemically, that is. One diet does not work for everybody nor do "one-size-fits-all" dosages of vitamins, minerals and amino acids. Every individual, because of unique genetic makeup, has distinct nutritional requirements that must be fulfilled in order to achieve and maintain optimal health and well-being. In fact, the concept of biochemical individuality was introduced by the renowned biochemist Roger Williams, PhD, nearly fifty years ago.

Today, the torch has been passed to Ellie Cullen.

As you will read in her groundbreaking book *Normal Blood Test Scores Aren't Good Enough!*, Ellie has perfected the interpretation of both standardized and specialized blood tests (the ones that access cardiovascular and cancer risk) to reveal each individual's unique pattern of health. In essence, your future health is contained within these pages. Her system can determine the current state of your health, track these patterns and provide practical solutions through diet and lifestyle changes along with supplementation. And, because she is meticulous about using the same reference laboratory for subsequent blood testing, Ellie can pinpoint exactly how efficiently the solutions are working.

Simply put, the blood doesn't lie.

You simply have to know, as Ellie has learned by tracking thousands of clients throughout her career, how to read blood tests by being aware of the optimal, not simply "normal" ranges for health, as well as your own "personal normal." For example, when I received my YFH (Your Future Health) results and nutritional interpretation, Ellie told me that my blood sugar reading of 81 was way too low...for me. In light of my other values and the history of diabetes that runs in the family, I needed to raise my fasting blood sugar—significantly!

What a surprise!

As a reactive hypoglycemic for years, I knew that low blood sugar was often a precursor to elevated blood sugar—or diabetes. For years, I had been diligently working to balance my blood sugar and truly thought that my value of 81 (the norm range being 60-109) was just fine. Ellie informed me that not only was my blood sugar a potential problem for me—leading to diabetes as well as immune dysfunction down the road—but that the primary supplement that I had been taking for blood sugar— chromium picolinate to be exact—was not as effective as the GTF (glucose tolerance factor) form of chromium.

How did she know this? From the results of daily blood testing using GTF chromium to balance blood sugar readings—that's how.

Ellie's system is not only extremely valuable in evaluating the current state of your health but is invaluable in uncovering the specific areas you need to work on as an individual, such as raising blood sugar (like me), lowering LDL (the bad cholesterol) and managing homocysteine (the recently discovered risk factor for heart disease).

After my own positive personal experiences using Ellie's revolutionary system, I can only suggest that you share this book with your family, your friends and your physician. The YFH System will enable you and your enlightened practitioner to analyze and track blood tests from a scientifically documented nutritional perspective. At the very least you will be able to ensure quality health for you and those you care about. You may even save a life someday.

Ann Louise Gittleman PhD, CNS
Author of the USA Today Bestseller *The Fat Flush Plan*

Contents

PART II
Case Studies on Blood Testing,

PART III

Protein

Liver

Complete Blood Count (CBC)

Cholesterol/Lipid Profile

White Blood Cell (WBC) Details/Manual Differential

Cancer

Thyroid

Special Tests

PART IV
Blood Tests to Track for Specific Illnesses

How Much Do You Already Know?

Before you read any further, take this simple quiz to see just how blood-test savvy you already are. The answers may surprise you!

1. Preventive blood testing can reveal diseases for which there are no physical symptoms.　　　　　T　　F

2. Laboratory "normal" reference ranges are set by a central medical agency, and are based on the latest medical research.　　　　　T　　F

3. When doing blood tests to prevent disease, it is more beneficial to have your blood tested by several different labs, in order to see a better "well-rounded" picture.
　　　　　T　　F

4. Preventive blood tests are ordered routinely by most doctors these days, and if ordered, will be covered by insurance and/or Medicare.　　　　　T　　F

5. Knowing your blood test history is one of the best early warning tools for detecting disease and illness.
　　　　　T　　F

6. It is best to have blood test scores that fall within the lab "normal" reference range at about the mid-point, not too high and not too low.　　　　　T　　F

7. It's impossible for someone with a serious disease to have 56 blood tests done and have all of the scores fall within the laboratory "normal" reference range.　　T　　F

8. People with the same blood type have identical nutritional needs.　　　　　T　　F

(Answers on the following page)

1

Answers

1. True: Please read chapter 8 to learn more.

2. False: Laboratory "normal" Reference Ranges are individually and subjectively set by each laboratory medical director. There is no universal standard. To learn how these ranges are established read chapter 6.

3. False: Actually testing with the same lab is *more* beneficial especially if you are tracking the test score trends because your results are being generated by the same equipment and with the same standards. If there is a change in the equipment or analysis, most reference labs will notify the doctor who ordered the test. More details can be found in chapter 6.

4. False: Preventive blood tests are ordered *less* frequently today due to cost containment. Insurance and/or Medicare will not usually cover these tests. See chapter 11.

5. True: Chapter 7 will give you more details.

6. False: Sometimes, as with sodium, it is best to score in the mid-range. Other times, as with zinc, it is best to score at the higher end. And most of the time, as with liver, it is best to score at the lower end.

7. False: YFH has many clients whose scores fall within the Lab "normal" Reference Range, yet they have cancer or various rare diseases. Read about Lena's Rare Disease in the case study section.

8. False: Nutritional needs, regardless of blood type, are unique to each individual. Accurate interpretation of results from extensive blood testing can reveal specific needs, and also help determine which foods need to be added or deleted from the basic group of foods. See chapter 12.

Introduction
Betty Kamen, PhD

This is a story of discovery—a finding so important, I believe it should be shouted from every rooftop. To say that it is about blood testing is not only an understatement, but hardly depicts the significance of what is chronicled in these pages.

Most of us have had our blood drawn and analyzed at one time or another. Few people go to the doctor for the purpose of prevention, so the familiar blood test is usually administered to confirm or deny your doctor's suspicions about your specific symptoms. If you are overweight or appear to have heart-related problems, the doctor will surely suggest a cholesterol check. If you complain of fatigue, then your iron levels, and perhaps your thyroid hormones are looked at. Using the results to graphically demonstrate your need for medical treatment, your doctor will point to test scores that are outside the "normal" range, and act according to standard protocol.

But he or she is unlikely to explain that the traditional parameters for health and disease, as established by these tests, are somewhat arbitrary—that they hardly reveal the entire story. Nor do most doctors explain terms like bilirubin, blood urea nitrogen, or alkaline phosphatase. They may not even offer a copy of the chart that pinpoints where you are on the grand scale of general results—unless you ask for it.

It is now common knowledge that the tiny constituents of your blood can only meet the intricate demands of your tissues and organs when nutrient makeup is optimum. The good news is that these minuscule blood cells contain coded messages that "file" this information. Better news is that the use of a high-tech microscope and a specially developed computer can expose these inner secrets—the ones that let us know whether or not nutrient needs are being met. But the effectiveness of the interpretations of these once elusive facts also depends on the skill of the scientists looking through the lens or examining the computer screen, and, most especially, of those who evaluate the very specific data that is as individual as your fingerprint.

And here's the important part: In addition to defining blood test terms and using the most highly professional analytical modalities, what Ellie Cullen offers is information about blood test scores that can give you feedback before a problem or its symptoms are noticed — well in advance of a time when interference with life quality, or even with life itself, becomes palpable.

Ellie tells a story that was twenty-five years in the making. What she discovered while analyzing endless blood tests is that there is almost always an avoidable cause for all disease. Such expert analysis is part of the innovative HealthPrint, now available to everyone. HealthPrint offers analysis that can "finger" a cells-out-of-order situation long before the usual blood test can. And then, following the gospel of tried-and-true measures, plus the very latest research, Ellie Cullen's scientific laboratory provides sound advice for helping to turn things around.

Normal Blood Test Scores Aren't Good Enough! is a fantastic resource—an invaluable tool for helping you to take control of your health with unrivaled precision. Keep in mind that your delicate blood cells are highly vulnerable and subject to ongoing change. And again—remember that the sleuthing detective work of the HealthPrint can discern malfunction at its earliest stages.

Betty Kamen, PhD
Medical Nutrition Reporter

Lose Weight with the California Calcium Countdown, Betty Kamen's 1,001 Health Secrets, She's Gotta Have It!: The Essential Sex Health Manual Every Woman Must Read and Hormone Replacement Therapy: How to Make an Informed Decision are among Dr. Kamen's 21+ popular books, described in detail at www.bettykamen.com.

"The doctor of the future will give no medicine but will interest his patients in the care of the human frame, in diet, in the causes of disease, and the prevention of disease."

Thomas Edison
(inventor of the phonograph and the electric light bulb, 1847-1931)

The Coming Age of Personalized Health

We're in the beginning stages of possibly the most revolutionary transformation of medical understanding of human biology in history.

It's an exciting time because, over the next few years, this transformation will make health, well-being and life without disease available to a much greater number of people than those who currently enjoy these greatest of gifts.

Most health and medical breakthroughs in the past have been predicated on the "sameness" of people. Antibiotics and the vast majority of drugs have been designed for, and given to, *everyone*. The FDA recommends one, and only one, universal nutrition plan. In neither case are differences such as age, gender, weight, height, genetics, environment, or biochemistry ever collectively considered.

This "one-size-fits-all" approach to health has been successful to some degree. Antibiotics have saved countless lives, and general nutrition guidelines have eliminated some of the worst afflictions related to dietary deficiencies. For example Rickets, a childhood disorder caused by vitamin D deficiency, is now rarely seen in the US because minimum daily requirements have been established for vitamin D for all ages.

But "one-size-fits-all" healthcare is the wrong approach for optimizing individual health and wellness.

People simply don't have the same biologies. Not every patient responds in like manner to the same drug. Doctors often practice trial and error to find the drugs that work best for each person and offer the fewest side effects.

On a personal level, who hasn't started the same diet with a friend or family member, only to find that one person loses weight easily, and the other isn't able to lose weight at all? And why do two people who live in the same environment, eat the same food, have the same stresses, age at different rates and catch different illnesses? Why does one person thrive on vigorous exercise, and another break down from it?

These differences exist because even though the essential "sameness" of our humanity allows most of us to benefit from penicillin and general-purpose nutritional recommendations, our individual biological differences need to be taken into account if we are to "optimize" our own personal health.

Thanks to recent scientific breakthroughs in molecular biology, the process of optimizing personal health is becoming easier. This innovative science makes it very clear that each of us is unique.

Understanding our common humanity took us quite far over the years to improve the overall health of our species. But the emerging knowledge of our biochemical uniqueness is taking us much farther—much faster. A few examples:

• In some cases, genetic tests have been designed to help doctors determine in advance which drugs will be most effective for individual patients, without the need for a lengthy and potentially dangerous trial and error process. (It may soon be possible to design personalized drugs that work especially well for a particular individual's genetic profile.)

• Profiling your unique set of genes will offer clues to your body's propensity for specific illnesses and diseases— allowing you to take preventive steps in advance. This will minimize the possibility of that disease or illness developing later in life.

• In the area of wellness, there's already one company, with doubtless many more to follow, designing personalized vitamins, based on an extensive individual survey questionnaire.

Peter D'Adamo's best-selling book, *Eat Right for Your Type*, offers a range of diets that address different nutritional needs resulting from specific blood types. A number of individuals have achieved great results by following blood-type-based nutrition plans. But shedding light on your blood type is only the beginning of what blood analysis can offer you. If you want to optimize your health, longevity, and weight control, blood analysis can help by customizing diet and lifestyle choices based on your own individual biochemistry.

This may come as a surprise to you. Almost everyone has had a blood test at one time or another, but other than being told that results were normal or not, you rarely are told anything at all about how your test results can be used to improve your health.

There's a reason for that. The vast majority of blood tests ordered by doctors are used only to confirm the presence of illness or disease. Blood testing works quite effectively for this.

But blood testing holds even greater promise because it can serve as a truly extraordinary tool for moving you up on the good-health continuum. Blood test results can be nutritionally analyzed and interpreted to develop a diet and wellness plan customized to your unique genes and biochemistry. This can only happen when blood testing is used preventively, rather than as a diagnostic tool after symptoms of illness or disease are already apparent.

Here's another way of expressing the difference between *symptom-driven* versus *preventive-driven* blood testing. Let's say you get an annual physical, and every year your blood sugar level rises a few points—but stays within a range that your doctor considers normal. The lab won't flag your score, and your doctor will probably tell you that you're normal—until a few years later when your score slips out of the normal range. At that point your doctor will tell you that you have adult onset diabetes, also known as Type 2 diabetes.

If your various blood sugar tests were being analyzed preventively, the ongoing rise in your scores would raise alarm bells, and your medical practitioner would be helping you make changes in your diet and lifestyle to prevent you from ever crossing the line into diabetes. Preventive blood testing tracks these potentially harmful movements out of optimal ranges.

For over two decades the company I founded and continue to run, Your Future Health (YFH), has been designing customized diet and wellness plans, based on comprehensive blood analysis, for a wide range of clients. This includes those seeking to overcome as well as prevent illness and disease.

Our clients' results have completely exceeded those which would have been possible on even the best general purpose diet and wellness plans. Therefore, many of our clients have asked me to put together a small, easy to read book to explain how to use blood testing to "individually" improve health.

In the following chapters, I'll attempt to do exactly that.

"Man is a food-dependent creature. If you don't feed him, he will die. If you feed him improperly, part of him will die."

Emanuel Cheraskin, MD, DMD
(Renowned Scientist and Educator, 1916-2001)

What Exactly Is Preventive Blood Testing?

Before getting into the details, I want to give you the big picture on what preventive blood testing is and how it works.

Let's talk for a moment about cholesterol. Your doctor tests your blood and tells you that your cholesterol level is too high. So he/she gives you recommendations for dietary changes that will help lower your cholesterol to a range considered optimal—usually less than 200. You follow these recommendations, and your next cholesterol blood test confirms that the changes you made to your diet succeeded in lowering your cholesterol level.

Or if these changes did not lower your cholesterol level, your doctor can use the results of the second test to fine-tune a new set of dietary suggestions that will probably work better for your particular biology. In either case, if you succeed in lowering your cholesterol, you'll succeed in reducing your risk of disease.

That's the essence of preventive blood testing.

The first step is a blood test to determine your current level for one or more parameters—such as cholesterol.

The second step is to make dietary or lifestyle changes based on your test results that will raise or lower your blood chemistry levels.

And the third step is to test again, to make certain that the changes you've made are working. If they aren't, the second test provides the information needed to make adjustments that will work better for you.

Most people know about cholesterol testing, but not too many people realize there is a vast range of additional blood parameters that can also be of great value to help prevent or to solve a variety of medical problems.

In our extensive clinical work, YFH has found that for most people between the ages of fifty-six and seventy, specific blood tests cover the essential parameters required for prevention, managing or treating disease. I provide details about each of these tests in later chapters.

But let's back up for a moment. What's the exact connection between preventive blood testing and improving your health? To avoid getting too bogged down in science, I'll simply explain what doctors and other health professionals have learned about the relationship between blood and overall health.

First, your blood reflects the current condition of virtually every aspect of your body. If you've got a cold, your blood analysis will reflect it. A consistent elevation of blood sugar is evidence of diabetes. There is literally nothing about your biological condition that your blood does not reveal.

Second, your blood chemistry reflects pending diseases well in advance of any symptoms. So regular, comprehensive blood testing allows emerging medical problems to be dealt with in the earliest, most treatable stages.

Third, when the parameters of your blood results aren't the best, you can almost always improve them through diet and vitamin supplements—that is, through nutrition. We cannot emphasize this point more strongly. We have seen, time and time again, that a nutritional program customized to each person's unique biochemistry is the most effective way to help prevent or solve just about every health problem. In extreme cases, medical treatment and drugs may be necessary, but the vast majority of our clients have responded quite well to dietary changes alone. A nutrition plan customized to each person's biochemistry (determined from blood analysis) very effectively balances the blood parameters which are most essential to good health. And once these parameters are within the *good-health* range, the body becomes strong enough to heal itself.

This is the heart of preventive blood testing.

YFH doesn't specialize in any one symptom area, but we've been able to help our clients and their doctors prevent or solve problems ranging from cancer to heart disease to digestive disorders. We have even been able to alleviate symptoms of infertility, diabetes and dozens of other afflictions.

You'll meet some of these people in the following pages as I explain details of preventive blood testing.

Blood Tests vs. Other Kinds of Medical Testing— Which Is Best?

There are a variety of different methods that can evaluate your biological systems. Why does YFH focus on blood tests? Because testing your blood gives the best possible mix of comprehensiveness, accuracy and affordability.

More specifically, blood tests have three main advantages when compared to other tests that evaluate biological systems. One, blood tests measure what is available to your cells now not what is left over as with urine samples. Two, by thorough blood testing one can zero in on a specific parameter (like cholesterol) or one can look at the interdependencies of several parameters (like cholesterol, triglycerides and glucose). Three, blood tests are respected by the medical community and, as such, are often used to justify the expense of further testing like MRI's, Cat Scans, ECG's and biopsies to insurance companies.

The typical way to test blood is to draw it from a vein in your arm. Another alternative is to stick the finger with a lancet and squeeze the blood into a tube. This method can be much less accurate. Squeezing your finger can alter cellular structures and, therefore, alter test results. For example, blood sugar and cholesterol levels are usually lower when blood is drawn from a finger rather than from a vein in your arm. In addition to being less accurate, when blood is drawn from the finger, there are fewer test categories.

Urine tests are invaluable for pH analysis which measure acidity and alkalinity levels, but are limited for testing overall health. There are numerous types of urine tests and they are generally considered reliable for heavy metals and drug testing. But these tests report only what is left over, not what is available now to live cells. In effect, they report old information.

Saliva tests are primarily used for testing hormones and are generally accurate although there is even some controversy here, too. They are of limited use in testing other parameters. Traditional MD's have more respect for hormone levels tested from a blood sample.

A new testing methodology of potential promise is computed tomography (CT) scanning—commonly known as full body 3-D scans. Working similarly to MRI's, CT scans "paint" a picture of your body's internal systems, and are able to spot tumors, blocked arteries and other potential health problems before the patient reflects any symptoms.

As to the effectiveness of CT's, the consensus among physicians is mixed, but YFH believes that CT systems, when used by a well-trained operator, work very well.

The main problem with CT scans is the high cost. A full set of body scans can cost $3,500 or more, and the fee is rarely covered by medical insurance. A comprehensive series of blood tests are able to reveal most of the same information at a fraction of the expense.

In my view, the most effective way to use a CT body scan is in tandem with blood testing. That is, first do a series of blood tests; and if those tests reveal any problems or areas needing further investigation, order the necessary body scans. Of course, if money is not a consideration, doing both the CT body scan and blood testing provides the most information.

But of the four testing procedures (urine, saliva, CT scans and blood tests), a comprehensive series of blood tests is of greater proven value, of broader scope, offers universal acceptance within the medical community, and is considerably more affordable.

Understanding Your Blood Type

Do you know your blood type? If so, do you know what makes the different blood types, well...different?

The simple answer is that blood is typed according to the antigens on the red blood cells. Antigens are substances that ellicit the formation of antibodies (protein molecules made by the immune system to neutralize foreign substances when introduced into the body.)

Type O has no antigens. It's formed from a long chain of repeating sugar molecules called fucose.

Type A has "A" antigens and is formed when fucose and another sugar called N-acetyl-galactosamine are combined.

Type B has "B" antigens and is formed when fucose and yet another sugar called D-galactose combine.

Type AB has both "A" and "B" antigens and is formed when fucose, N-acetyl-galactosamine, and D-galactose combine.

But this simple chemical explanation only tells us that not all blood is the same, and that based on type, O blood can be universally donated to all other blood types, and AB types can accept blood from all other blood types.

It is theorized that the four different blood types evolved under different conditions, and that we don't do well with foods that were not a part of that particular evolution. For more explicit details of this theory, refer to the research of Dr Peter J. D'Adamo.[1]

Type O is the oldest evolved blood type, and the most common worldwide. Those with O blood tend to have rugged immune and digestive systems that evolved over millennia, most probably when early mankind lived mainly on a diet of meat. In our clinical work, we've found that type O individuals tend to respond best to high protein diets including meat, poultry, and fish, as well as to fruits and vegetables. Grains, legumes and dairy products appear to be less suited to those with O blood.

Type A is the next oldest blood type, theorized to have emerged between 25,000 and 15,000 years BC—at a time when agriculture was evolving. At YFH, we've found that

---

[1] If you're interested in blood type and diet, you may want to read Peter D'Adamo's *Eat Right For Your Type*. Additionally, the YFH HealthPrint Guide also covers blood-type based diets. But, the food recommendations not only consider blood type but enumerate the high carbohydrate and high glycemic foods for every category.

type A clients tend to thrive on a vegetarian diet where most of the protein comes from plant sources. Type A's can usually eat grains with no problems, and fish suits type A's better than meat or poultry.

Type B blood probably emerged between 15,000 and 10,000 years BC, during a time when nomads roamed the landscape, living off their domestic livestock. We've found that type B's can usually thrive on the most varied diets, including meats, dairy products, fruits, vegetables, and grains.

Type AB blood is presumed to have emerged only ten to fifteen centuries ago, and is the rarest category type. We've found that the best diet for AB's is primarily vegetarian, with small amounts of meat and dairy.

You may have heard that blood also has a positive or negative factor called Rh factor. Eighty percent of humans have positive Rh. Twenty percent have negative Rh factor present on the surface of the cell. This is important when receiving a transfusion or during childbirth but does not appear to impact dietary needs.

Your blood type and your diet are directly related to optimum health, as there are real differences in the way different people respond, even to something as innocuous as a glass of milk.

We also bring up blood type because, as mentioned earlier, a number of YFH clients have achieved very good health results by following a blood-type based diet. The specific foods that individuals of each blood type should eat and the research both go well beyond the scope of this book.[1]

You should be aware, however, that regardless of blood type, a diet of totally pure organic raw foods will improve one's health. Sometimes following the specific foods for your blood type is not as important as correcting nutrient imbalances and avoiding foods that are high in carbohydrates and high on the glycemic index.

Eating the proper foods for your blood type is only scratching the surface when looking at how to optimize health. In the same way that humanity has evolved with different blood types, your own genetic biochemical makeup is the result of evolution. You are predisposed to specific nutritional and lifestyle choices under which you will thrive. And the way to find out what will work best for you is to have your blood analyzed.

> "The greatest discovery of any generation is that human beings can alter their lives by altering the attitudes of their minds."
>
> **Albert Schweitzer**
> **(German physician and philosopher, 1875-1965)**

All Blood Tests Are
Not Created Equal

There are hundreds upon hundreds of different types of blood tests. One medical guide lists over seven hundred separate tests, and that guide is far from complete.

To make matters even more confusing, there are a variety of tests to evaluate identical factors. And different sets of equipment for the same test can yield dissimilar results or conclusions based on different scales. As we'll discuss later, different labs have their own way of determining what that particular lab considers a normal result.

In the past you didn't have to worry about any of these details. You simply went to your doctor, and he or she knew how to get the best, most accurate and most useful blood test results. But in this era, it's important to know more about your own medical and preventive treatments. Medical insurance programs are beginning to cover fewer procedures and tests, and chances are you no longer have only one doctor you've known for years, the doctor who knows your complete medical history. These days we're obligated to play a leading role in our own medical and preventive health.

So how do you know what tests to order, and if those tests are being done properly? Here are a few suggestions.

First, make sure that the laboratory doing the processing is what the blood testing industry calls a *reference lab*. A reference lab is used by other labs to provide a definitive answer to questionable results, or to process rarely ordered and expensive tests that regular blood labs do not have the equipment and/or the expertise to perform. They have the most skilled personnel, the newest and best processing equipment, and are at the cutting edge of testing protocols.

There are thousands of blood labs in the country, and only a few are reference labs. Are other blood labs bad? Not at all. But in our years of clinical practice, we've always found that the additional expertise to skillfully handle the full range of essential blood tests make it worthwhile and cost effective to work only with reference labs. Your health, after all, is priceless; and if you're going to base significant diet and lifestyle changes on a set of numbers provided by a blood lab, you should feel confident that those numbers are accurate.

Always try to do your regular annual or semi-annual blood testing with the same lab. The same protocol and equipment should be used if possible to ensure the greatest accuracy. That way the results you get should be directly comparable to previous results.

If you test at different labs, even if you order the same exact tests, the procedures, scales, and even normal ranges can differ, precluding easy comparability of results over time. If you always try to test at the same lab, you'll avoid this problem provided that the lab you choose, or the company who oversees your results, keeps you informed regarding any equipment changes. Equipment changes could influence the lab normal reference range of the tests you are comparing.

Find out what sort of interpretive guide comes with the lab results you'll receive. Getting the right set of properly executed blood tests is essential, but you will also need a set of guidelines that explain your results and then tell you what you need to know to improve your scores.

Finally, you'll need to know the ideal target range for each parameter of your blood test results. This is so important that we've devoted the next chapter to the question of blood test ranges.

When you begin to have your blood tested, make sure to follow these guidelines:

1. **Have your blood tested at a reference lab.**
2. **Use the same lab analysis center for all your tests.**
3. **Make sure you get a clear and concise interpretative guide along with your results.**
4. **Learn the ideal target range for each result.**

"The natural force within each one of us is the greatest healer of disease, let your food be your medicine."

Hippocrates
(Father of Medicine, 460?-377? BC)

What's Normal for a Blood Test? And How Is It Determined?

When your doctor tells you that the result of one of your blood tests is "normal," what exactly does that mean?

If you're like most people, you just assume that it means that you're doing fine for that particular test—that there are no problems. If you think about it at all, you probably assume that the *normal* range is something that the specialists have determined to be the *right* range. In other words, normal might be considered the ideal range, or at least a range that's good enough.

In fact, nothing could be farther from the truth. To understand why, it's necessary to learn where lab normal ranges come from. Your blood test report usually lists the name of the test, your score, and then the upper and lower limits of lab "normal" reference range for that particular test. If your score is out of the normal range, it's usually flagged in some way to draw attention to it.[2]

So where does the lab get its data on normal ranges? In most cases, the lab director sets the normal range, and the procedure he or she uses to set the range can vary widely.

Originally, normal blood ranges were set by taking a large representative sample of healthy members of a population, testing them, and charting the results in the shape of a bell. At the high point on the bell curve—that is, the point that represents the majority of the tested population, a standard deviation is determined setting the high normal and low normal values. And that range is considered the lab normal reference range. Note that "normal" means the range of the *majority*, which is not necessarily either good or bad. Normal is often confused with average.

Some labs differentiate normal ranges on the basis of gender and age, but few consider weight, height or other parameters, that may be very significant.

It is now fairly common for blood labs to determine normal ranges by averaging the results from the patients who have been tested by that lab. They often also use scores from insurance and pre-surgery testing, and they take into account suggestions from the equipment manufacturers. In all cases, whether using a broad population or only the clients of a particular lab, it's easy to see that these methods for determining laboratory normal reference ranges are extremely problematic, and can vary greatly.

---

[2] Your result can be out of the normal range either because it is worse than normal, or because it is better than normal.

The first problem is that labs can and do have different ranges that they consider normal. So it's possible to have the same test result evaluated as normal and abnormal by two different labs.

An obvious problem in using clients of a lab for the control group to determine a normal range is that the majority of people having their blood tested are doing so because they have symptoms of a medical problem. So they can be expected to have blood results which are not normal for healthy people. That throws off the normal calculation.

Does that mean you should only use a blood lab that determines its lab normal reference ranges from results of healthy population averages? Unfortunately, even with averages from healthy populations, there's still a problem.

Here's why: In the US, obesity affects more than fifty percent of our population, and this percentage has been increasing steadily over the years. Obesity negatively skews a wide range of blood chemistry values. Diabetes, which has reached epidemic proportions in this country, largely as a result of obesity, does the same.

Because both conditions (obesity and diabetes) are becoming more common, one might expect that a statistical sample from a population control group taken currently would yield a broader range of results than a similar test performed thirty years ago (that is, during a time when fewer people were obese or had diabetes). This is in fact true. Blood ranges for a number of key tests are widening as obesity and other conditions escalate. The average American isn't as healthy now as he or she was thirty years ago, and blood results reflect this.

Instead of interpreting this increasing unhealthiness as a red flag indicating that our overall population needs to get its dietary and lifestyle act together, the majority of blood labs have broadened the ranges that they consider "normal." And in a sense, these broader ranges *are* normal since they continue to represent the top of the bell curve of population average ranges. These new wider ranges are definitely not optimum, because they are based on averages of people who are not in the best of health.

A final problem with the standard range of normal blood results is that what may be optimum for one person may not be for another.

More than two decades of clinical work confirmed for YFH that blood ranges vary according to age, gender, weight, and height. A twenty-something, two-hundred-pound, six-foot-four male linebacker doesn't have the same set of optimum ranges as a seventy-something, ninety-five pound, five-foot-four grandmother.

Individual biochemistry is far too complex to determine ideal normal ranges for any one person solely on the basis of categories. To fully interpret these ranges, it's essential to determine a *personal* normal range, which is unique to each of us.

And I'll explain exactly how to do this in the next chapter.

> "The art of healing comes from nature and not from the physician. Therefore, the physician must start from nature with an open mind."
>
> Paracelsus
> (Swiss Physician, 1493-1541)

Determining Your Personal
Normal Blood Ranges

The more precisely you determine what your body needs for health and wellness, the easier it is to achieve it. Since the 1970's, YFH has been tabulating the tightest possible blood range levels that have worked best for our clients according to age, gender, height and weight. We've accumulated more than twenty years of data from thousands of clients, effectively completing one of the largest—if not the largest—clinical trials in the country for optimum blood results broken down by the categories cited above. As validated by many physicians, our data on optimum blood ranges may be the best available.

So why not list these ranges here? One of the greatest benefits we could provide is to let you know the goals that you should be attempting to achieve. Right?

Right, but unfortunately, to provide that data here would be difficult at best, and misleading at worst.

Difficult because of the amount of data we'd need to list. YFH has developed good-health ranges for a few hundred blood parameters. For most of our clients, we track between fifty-six and seventy specific levels. Specifying data by gender, age, height and weight means that we have thousands of possible optimum ranges, depending on each client's biological characteristics.

Misleading because we cannot control the consistency or accuracy of other blood labs. As mentioned earlier, different blood labs use different scales for tabulating results, divergent ways of testing the same sample, and different protocols for preparing the sample for analysis.

The fact is that our optimum blood ranges would not necessarily correlate to blood tests completed elsewhere, just as the ranges of other labs would not correlate with ours.

But the biggest reason that we can't simply list optimum ranges here is that these values can change as your other test scores change. For example, calcium, magnesium and phosphorous vary in relationship to each other.

In the next chapter, I'll tell you more about your *Personal Normal*—why knowing your own Personal Normal is one of the most powerful health tools ever developed.

"When health is absent, wisdom cannot reveal itself, art cannot become manifest, strength cannot be expected, wealth is useless, and reason is powerless."

Herophilies
(Physician to Alexander the Great, 300 BC)

Testing Your Blood Over Time:
The Holy Grail of Preventive Health

In the last chapter, we discussed the benefits of continually narrowing the categories into which your own biochemistry falls. But optimum health comes when you narrow things down so tightly that no one but *you* is in the category—a category of one, which represents your own unique biochemistry.

How great is the value of doing this? In my own case, and in the case of many of my clients, it may have been the difference between life and death. More on this in a moment. First I want to explain how to determine your own category of one; that is, how to determine your own Personal Normal.

To determine your own personal normal ranges, you should have a comprehensive blood test every year, or ideally every six months. If you have a specific medical problem, you may want to test as often as every three months, as do many of our clients.

Each time you test, examine your results, and make changes that will bring your scores into the optimum ranges that are specific to your biology. The YFH test provides an extensive guide that tells you how to do this. Other health practitioners may have different methods to improve your scores.

If you follow these guidelines, your scores should improve. In addition to the improvement, you'll see that there are some results with unchanging values, particularly if you began testing preventively, rather than as a way of solving a particular medical problem. Barring a specific medical problem or extremely inconsistent lifestyle and diet, most, if not all, of your scores will tend toward a particular level.

For example, your optimum target range for a white blood cell test called *Bands* may be between zero and two. Anywhere within that range may be excellent for those of your gender and approximate age, height and weight. Let's say that in testing four times you always have a score between zero and one. If so, your score between zero and one is your Personal Normal for Bands. Someone else, after multiple tests over time, may have a Personal Normal of three to four. These two different Personal Normals could be ideal for each of you if both scores are within the general range for your respective genders, ages, height and weight.

Each person has a Personal Normal range for every blood test parameter, and each range is determined exactly the same way as it was for the Bands test. All of your Personal Normal scores are the key to fully understanding and managing your current and future health.

Why is that? What's the specific benefit of knowing your Personal Normal blood ranges?

In a nutshell, it's the single best early warning tool for preventing and/or identifying disease and illness before they get established in your system. It's a way of preventing disease or knocking it out in the earliest, most treatable stage—the stage when therapy has the greatest chance of success. It's also the best way to keep your own unique biological system operating at its best.

I mentioned earlier that knowing my Personal Normal scores, and specifically, my Personal Normal Bands score, probably saved my life. I'd like to tell you about that experience.

A few years ago, I had a routine blood test. My Bands score was a nine. My Personal Normal for Bands had always been between zero and one. Since the lab normal range for Bands is usually considered to be between zero and ten, a Bands score of nine is within the lab normal range. Most doctors would have considered my score as an indication that nothing was wrong. After all, I was in the lab normal range, and didn't exhibit any symptoms that were out of the ordinary. In fact, this was exactly what my dermatologist told me. In his opinion, I was fine.

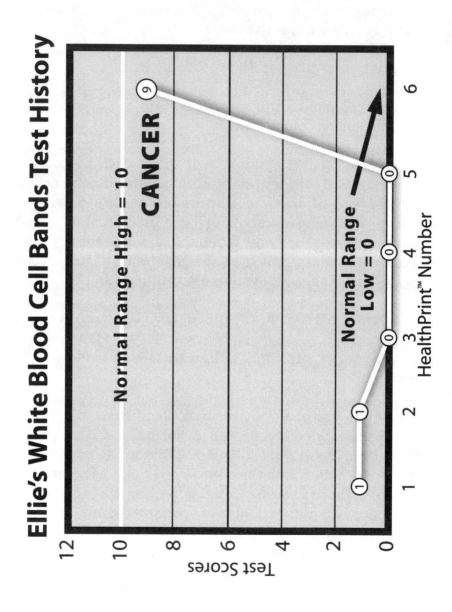

Ellie's White Blood Cell Bands Test History

But take a look at the graph (on the previous page) of my Bands tests over the past few years. Does a score of nine look normal for me? **No!**

At YFH, time and time again we see that dramatic movements from established Personal Normal scores are virtually always an early warning sign of a developing problem. In the case of Bands, an increasing score may mean one of two things: 1) The person taking the test has a cold or disease weakening his or her immune system. Or, 2) the person taking the test has skin cancer or an impending skin abnormality that may develop into skin cancer.

I hadn't been sick, so I insisted that my dermatologist do a second, much more thorough exam. And lo and behold! He found a small cancerous patch on my arm that he removed before it could spread. This particular form of cancer is fast acting and potentially lethal. That I caught it so early almost certainly saved my life.

Without an established Personal Normal range for Bands, neither my doctor nor I would have had any idea at all that I had skin cancer—until I developed symptoms. And by then it may have been too late.

I mentioned in the earliest pages of this book that virtually every forthcoming medical problem is reflected in your blood chemistry in advance of any symptoms or any decline in how you feel. A single blood test can help identify a wide range of problems early. But for the ultimate in advance warning, and to be able to identify the widest possible range of potential and/or forthcoming medical problems, there is simply no substitute for establishing Personal Normal blood ranges by testing regularly over time. I consider this of paramount importance.

> **For the ultimate in advance warning of any forthcoming medical problems, there is simply no substitute for establishing Personal Normal blood ranges by testing regularly with the same system over time.**

Beyond preventing disease, there are additional benefits for establishing your Personal Normal ranges, discussed in the next two chapters.

"The superior physician helps before the early budding of disease . . . To administer medicines to diseases which have already developed is comparable to the behavior of those persons who begin to dig a well after they have become thirsty."

Huang Ti
(Chinese Emperor, 2697 - 2597 BC)

Why Your Doctors Can't Order Your Full Range of Blood Tests... Even When They Want To

It's said that in ancient Chinese villages, the villagers paid the doctor when they were well. If they became sick, the doctor failed, so the villagers stopped payment until they became well again.

This is virtually the reverse of worldwide practice today. If you think about it, it's very sensible to direct medical resources more to the prevention of illness than its treatment. We all want to avoid getting sick rather than going through the process of recovering from an illness.

Nevertheless, for all the vaunted abilities of Western medicine, our entire health apparatus is far from ideal when it comes to early detection and prevention of disease.

Our American health establishment has the best diagnostic equipment in the world. Those who live abroad

41

and can afford it, check into our greatest research hospitals for cutting edge treatments in cardiology and a range of other specialties. The primary focus, however, is *fixing* problems and not *preventing* them.

Why aren't our *preventive* health programs the best in the world?

American medical practice tends to be predicated on the idea that if you're not sick, you're well. Assuming that health is the absence of illness and disease has vast implications about the way we think about wellness. And it determines the medical institutions we develop to serve our needs. When a society considers health the absence of illness, it tends to begin medical treatments at the point illness begins, since it assumes there isn't a problem until that time.

YFH could not disagree more. Heart disease, cancer, diabetes and the vast majority of health challenges that are epidemic take decades to become noticeable. But YFH has seen firsthand that predictive changes in blood chemistry usually happen well in advance of the advent of symptoms.

Understanding the difference between the premise that health is the absence of illness, and that health is something you need to achieve, is the first step—both individually and as a society—for optimizing health. There are a few more down-to-earth, brass-tack explanations for why we, as a society, aren't particularly good at preventive health.

Prevention is perceived as too expensive, offering less potential profit than treatment, and the system that governs how medical resources are deployed works against prevention—even when doctors try to support preventive health initiatives.

If you're like most people, it probably seems absurd that preventing illness would be more expensive than treating it. But if you view it from the perspective of medical insurance companies, it starts to make some sense.

Cancer is a good example. There are a range of tests that can predict cancer growth well in advance of the advent of symptoms. If everyone took this set of tests, the vast majority of cancer cases would be caught much earlier, and treatment would be more effective and less expensive.

But from a medical insurer's perspective, it costs less overall to provide more expensive treatment to the relatively few persons who eventually develop cancer than it does to incur the larger expense of testing everyone repeatedly over time. The medical insurance industry in the US is made up mainly of companies in private industry, and these companies are expected to turn a profit. So it isn't surprising that they work to maximize revenues—and that means widespread (ultimately more expensive) preventive health programs get short-changed. YFH would argue that if everyone were tested for the most prevalent degenerative diseases, the cost would be less than the fully allocated cost of lost work time and treatment. For better or worse, a profit-driven health care system, though generating many benefits, places unfortunate limits on preventive health.

Another reason our society is not focused on prevention is that the primary components of preventive health are rarely a part of medical school curriculi. Until just a few years ago, courses on nutrition were rarely taught. Consequently, many doctors did not learn about long-term methods to keep people from getting sick.

Again, our beliefs about health determine the institutions that our society creates to serve its needs. Thus our medical industry, across the board, is very treatment, rather than prevention, oriented. And this is why your doctor doesn't generally order all the blood tests that we at YFH have determined to be essential for optimum health.

If you go to your doctor and ask for a panel of blood tests, your doctor will likely ask you what symptoms you're experiencing. If you indicate that you want tests for preventive health reasons, you will probably be told that the blood tests can't be justified for reimbursement from the HMO, insurance company, or from Medicare without a specific problem or symptom.

Some doctors may also advise that preventive blood testing is a waste of time and money—that if you feel fine, you're fine. It's for this reason that the majority of blood tests in the US are ordered only after the onset of medical symptoms.

I don't want to criticize the American medical establishment or physicians. I am simply pointing out why doctors, HMO's, medical insurance and Medicare are not the place to look for affective means of preventive health. To prevent disease, the service of preventive blood testing becomes our personal responsibility, as is buying vitamins and making nutritional changes.

The good news is that this situation is in the process of changing. Growing numbers of doctors view nutrition, lifestyle choices and other aspects of preventive health as complementary to traditional medical care.

Along with forward-thinking physicians, we at YFH look at prevention as naturally complementary. Do everything you can to stay healthy, but do not avoid going to a doctor you trust—especially if your blood test results indicate a problem, or if you develop symptoms of illness or disease.

Next I want to share with you a little known, but troubling institution—whose existence prompts me to advise you to do your preventive blood testing confidentially, instead of through your insurance or Medicare provider.

"Real knowledge is to know the extent of one's ignorance."

Confuscius
(Chinese Philosopher, 551?-479? BC)

The Medical Information Bureau and Other Matters of Confidentiality

Have you ever heard of the Medical Information Bureau (MIB)? If you're like most people, you have not. The MIB is like a credit reporting agency for the insurance industry. But instead of tracking financial information, the MIB accumulates and tracks medical information. This information is then made available to MIB member companies—that is, to health, life and other insurance companies—if and when they request a medical report about you. "Member (insurance) companies submit information to the MIB in the form of codes. This information is obtained directly from insurance applicants—from doctors, hospitals, and medical or medically related facilities. Individuals applying for life, health, disability, or long-term care insurance from an MIB member company, give their consent during the underwriting process. These codes are reflective of the individual's medical history, avocations, and other risk factors."

So if you've ever applied for health or life insurance—and in many cases, even if you have not—you may have routinely given your consent for the MIB to gather information about your confidential medical history. You may have signed a release of information form, whenever you had a medical treatment or test, or when you applied for insurance.

It isn't hard to see the benefit of a centralized depository of medical information to insurance companies—and for that matter, to many of their clients. The more medical information these firms have access to, the more accurately they can set and differentiate their rates, and reduce insurance fraud. Healthy clients would receive lower rates, as they would be less likely to subsidize the higher claims costs of those with pre-existing conditions, dangerous hobbies, or genetic propensities for certain diseases.

Overall, insurance firms would be able to predict and quantify their claims costs, lowering their overall cost of operations. In the US, insurance, like medical care, is provided by private industry, so for better or worse, it's a strategic objective for insurance firms to make a profit in addition to providing good service to their clients. There's nothing wrong with that.

But there are potential problems with a centralized repository of medical information when the unwitting providers of that information may not even know it exists.

One of our clients had a substantial rate increase for his company's entire medical insurance program. After some investigation, it turned out that the owner's MIB file had mistakenly listed him as having diabetes, which, due to the estimated expense of treatment, caused the company's entire medical premiums to go up substantially. The owner was able to correct the information in his MIB file, but it took considerable time and expense.

We've heard of another case where a misdiagnosis that was subsequently corrected by a second diagnosis ended up in an MIB file, and again, only came to the knowledge of the person in question when his medical insurance rates increased.

So one problem with MIB files is that they may not have correct information about you, and unless you check your file regularly, there's no mechanism for correcting faulty data. Since most people don't even know such a file exists, a large number of these files are not being checked for accuracy.

A second problem relates exclusively to preventive medical testing. If, for example, you develop disease symptoms, it isn't unreasonable that your test results become part of your medical record—as long as you know about it.

But let's say that you feel fine, and you get tested for preventive reasons, yet results indicate that you may be at risk for a disease. What happens if that purely preventive blood test you took becomes part of your MIB file, and as a result of the suggested risk factor, your insurance is cancelled or your rates are raised? Isn't that penalizing you unjustly for having gone the added mile to prevent the very disease that would cost your insurance company considerable additional expense?

Worse, data reported to the MIB as a result of preventive tests that indicate that you are healthy can have highly negative repercussions on your medical and life insurance. One of our clients had a liver scan done for prevention, and her test results were excellent. When she tried to change her health insurance, she was turned down by a number of companies. When she attempted to find out why, a sympathetic person at one of the companies told her that her MIB file indicated that she'd had a liver scan. She protested that her test result was excellent. Nevertheless, she was told that it was the company's policy to decline coverage for anyone who had ever had a liver scan, regardless of the test outcome.

Obviously, companies that decline coverage base this policy on the assumption that anyone who gets a liver scan does so because they may have had a serious medical problem.

Because virtually all of our clients demand confidentiality, YFH never has, and never will, release client blood test results to anyone other than the client. We've found that there are a variety of legitimate reasons that people wish to keep their medical data confidential, and we are respectful of this. There are certainly other blood testing facilities that also offer confidential testing, but medical practitioners are generally required to provide their patients' information to the MIB if they accept insurance. Because YFH accepts neither insurance nor Medicaid, we are exempt from this requirement and are able to protect our clients' confidentiality.

If you don't wish your preventive test results to be made public, check with your doctor, testing company or lab to make sure that they don't release your results to MIB or elsewhere, especially if you pay for these tests yourself. The insurance companies usually feel that if they pay for your tests, they have a right to the data.

You may want to ask for this assurance in writing and that a notation is made on your file. The confidentiality of your test results may be assured if you test with a physician or lab that never releases any client data to MIB.

The second step you can take is to be sure you don't sign the consent forms that grant the right to release your test results. This consent is usually included with the general materials that health care providers routinely ask you to sign. Not signing this consent may be easier said than done. In some cases, medical care may only be provided if the form is signed. If it's important to keep your medical data confidential, give more than the usual cursory glance at these forms, and ask that the release-of-data section be crossed out.

The third step is to check your MIB file. Doing so is no more trouble than checking your credit reporting agency file.

1. Send a letter to the MIB requesting the forms to release a copy of your file to you. Be sure to include your return address. The letter should be sent to:

Medical Information Bureau
P.O. Box 105
Essex Station
Boston, MA 02112
617-426-3660

2. The MIB will send you a release form—their attempt to reduce the number of record requests. They usually include a letter assuring you that their records are accurate. This letter is in no way legally binding for the MIB, and should simply be ignored.

3. Send the completed form and required payment back to the MIB.

4. The MIB will either forward you a copy of your file, along with information about what to do if you find errors—or they will let you know that they don't maintain a file on you.

You can also go to the MIB's website and order your file directly.

www.mib.com

In the next chapter I'll tell you how preventive blood testing can dramatically increase the tests and medical procedures that your insurance firm will be willing to cover.

Winning at the Medical Insurance Game

I mentioned earlier that we at YFII consider preventive blood testing and medical treatment entirely complementary. Preventive blood testing provides doctors with the diagnostic horsepower to approve a wide range of additional tests and procedures for you. For example, when your blood tests indicate signs of disease before symptoms are evident, you can provide your doctor with results he or she needs to justify ordering additional tests and treatment which can be covered by your insurance plan or Medicare, and would not otherwise be covered.

Literally dozens of our clients have had everything from additional specialists, to surgery and MRI's paid for by their medical insurance companies as a direct result of the blood testing they've done with us. How did it work? Here are a few examples.

When we first met Ginni, she was deathly ill with Hepatitis C, and was under the care of a gamut of doctors. She'd had her blood evaluated several times before, but she had not been tested for the comprehensive series of blood panels that YFH includes—the kind that are rarely available elsewhere. After recovering from Hepatitis C with the help of YFH, Ginni began regular testing to prevent further disease. On one of her successive tests, she discovered an elevation for an ovarian cancer test (CA 125). Although this is a very controversial test in the medical profession, her doctor realized the value of this test after reviewing Ginni's upward trend rising from 20 to 55. This trend justified more testing (paid by insurance). And the additional ultrasound tests identified a benign (non-cancerous) ovarian tumor.

After repeating ultrasound and CA 125 tests during the next two months, it became clear that Ginni had a fast-growing benign ovarian tumor the size of an orange, that could rupture at any time. Therefore, surgery was required to remove the tumor. At the time of her surgery, Ginni still had no pain or symptoms. Because Ginni did this simple cancer test with her own money, she not only saved her life, but also reaped the benefit of more than $18,000 of extra medical costs that were covered by her insurance.

The following is another example of how preventive blood tests help get additional procedures covered by insurance—even when the blood test results were within the lab normal ranges.

Elizabeth had her HealthPrint done with YFH every four months for four years. One particular analysis called the Alkaline Phosphatase test saved her life. Each time she had this test done, her score ranged from 47 to 63 until the twelfth time, when her score jumped to 115. (See illustration on next page.) Elizabeth did not feel differently, and her score was within the laboratory normal range of 40 to 140. However, she was concerned about this sudden elevation, and took her trend of scores to her doctor. He said that since he could find no symptoms of a problem, she was fine. Elizabeth, however, felt that this was so unusual that she persuaded her doctor to order additional tests. These tests showed bone cancer in its earliest stages.

Not only did this prolong her life, her doctor was able to submit these additional tests totaling over $5,000.00 to Medicare for payment. Remember, the protocol for medical treatment in the US currently is not prevention-oriented. To justify tests you usually need to exhibit some sort of symptom. Elizabeth had no symptoms—only a blood test with a normal result that was not normal for her. If she waited until she was exhibiting symptoms, the cancer would have spread and may have been impossible to treat.

It's nice to know that the relatively small investment of preventive blood testing once or twice a year can have such benefits. If you don't find anything wrong, then you have the satisfaction of additional peace of mind. And if you do find something abnormal, the modest cost of a blood test can be the critical element that allows your HMO or insurance company to cover the cost of much more expensive tests and procedures—with the ultimate benefit to you of treatment in the earliest, most potentially successful stage.

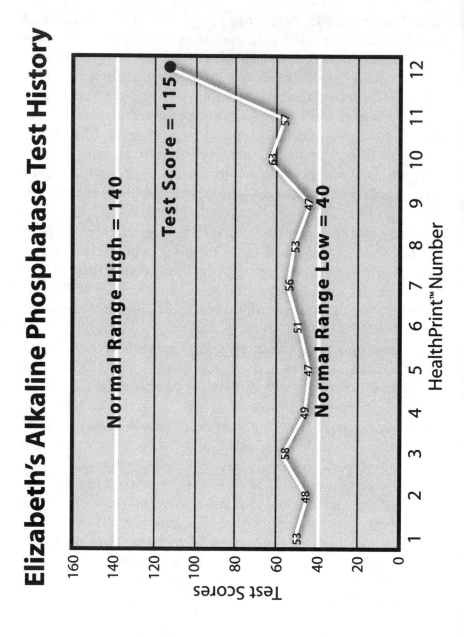

Elizabeth's Alkaline Phosphatase Test History

Normal Range High = 140

Test Score = 115

Normal Range Low = 40

HealthPrint™ Number

Test Scores

Once again, please remember that taking control of our health to prevent illness is our responsibility. Our doctors, insurance companies and Medicare are doing their part. But the job is too big—we need to help out and budget for these critical tests at least yearly. I, for instance, only have catastrophic insurance coverage to reduce my premiums, but I spend the savings on regular preventive testing.

More ways to save money while improving your health through regular blood testing are discussed next.

"A man may esteem himself happy when that which is his food is also his medicine."

Henry David Thoreau
(American Author, 1817-1862)

Optimum Health at Minimum Cost

We're lucky to live in an era that offers a vast range of dietary and lifestyle choices that promise increased wellness and disease prevention.

But the downside of so many options is that we have a bewildering array of decisions to make, and even worse, many of the most widespread and popular healthcare suggestions contradict other proposed choices.

For example, our federal government has told us for years that we should cut fat and cholesterol from our diet and replace them mainly with complex carbohydrates. Millions of people have done exactly that—trading eggs and bacon at breakfast for a bowl of cereal and skimmed milk. This advice continues to be offered by numerous respected caregivers as the most heart and cancer protective way of eating.

But is it really? One of the country's most well known cardiologists, Dr. Robert Atkins, believed that an overabundance of carbohydrates tends to lead to adult onset diabetes, which in turn is terrible for the heart. Dr. Atkins made the point that diabetes in this country is exploding, seemingly in tandem with increased reliance on the carbohydrate-heavy diets that Americans are now eating. His books recommend a low-carbohydrate diet, and tells his millions of followers to eat as much protein and fat as they wish. He even recommends a near one-hundred-percent fat diet for "metabolically resistant" persons who aren't able to lose weight on his suggested normal low-carbohydrate diet. "The first thing you will learn is that 900 calories of fat (90 percent of the 1000-calorie allotment) is provided by 100 grams of fat—not a lot of food."[3] Therefore, a small portion of fat provides a lot of calories.

Dr. Atkins considered a high-carbohydrate diet dangerous. Many other diet consultants consider a low-carbohydrate diet dangerous.

Another area of controversy is the proper dosage for supplements. The FDA's Minimum Daily Adult Requirement for a wide range of nutrients is only a small fraction of what many other health experts recommend. For example, Nobel Prize laureate Dr. Linus Pauling considered 5,000 to 10,000 mgs of vitamin C per day necessary for optimum health. On the other hand, the FDA suggests less than 100 mgs per day. Who's right?

---

[3] Robert C. Atkins, M.D., *Dr. Atkins New Diet Revolution*, New York: Bantam Books, 1972, p. 235

Actually, all of these experts may be right for some people, but no one program is right for everyone. The best way to know what is in *your* best health interest is through a nutritional interpretation of a comprehensive series of blood tests.

While health experts can disagree about the best diet and lifestyle choices, there is much less disagreement about the value of a comprehensive analysis of your blood to accurately reflect the real-time status of your health. So blood testing provides a great feedback mechanism for evaluating the effect of changes you've made. Hence blood testing lets you sort through all the contradictory health claims you hear, and know for certain which ones work best for you.

It might surprise you to know how different people react to the same health choices. Some of our clients need extremely high doses to register even a small improvement in their blood level range. Other clients would be risking their health with such large doses because they have more efficient absorption.

So in answer to the question of the proper dosage for supplements, the valid answer is: *it depends*. Blood testing is not the only way, but it could be the best way. No other method is as simple or offers a similar level of precision for determining your optimal levels.

Our clients' blood test results even demonstrate that some people achieve better health by using certain brands or formulations of supplements. For example, to eliminate asthma symptoms, one of our clients used magnesium chelate. When he switched to a magnesium oxide formulation, his asthma returned and his level of magnesium decreased. In each case, the identical number of milligrams was consumed. Therefore, our client learned that the chelated form was the best for him.

Many of our clients gradually increased their intake to dozens of nutrients a day as they continually heard about the positive health effects of the latest and greatest daily "supplement du jour." After doing a HealthPrint, many found out that quite a few of their regular daily supplements were neither necessary nor effective. Others discovered that their dosage levels for some supplements were either too high or too low. In general, the fine-tuning of supplementation through blood testing improved the effectiveness of those they continued to take, while eliminating the cost of others they didn't need. As an aside, YFH offers suggestions about supplement quality and formulations. However, YFH does not sell any supplements.

A number of forward thinking vitamin companies are already looking at individual client blood testing to prove the effectiveness of their product lines. Customizing supplements by blood chemistry analysis is almost certain to become the wave of the future.

In the next chapter, I discuss the blood testing analysis and nutritional recommendations that YFH put together in an inexpensive, easy to follow package that helps its clients achieve optimum health.

"I believe that you can, by taking some simple and inexpensive measures, extend your life and your years of well-being. My most important recommendation is that you take vitamins every day in optimum amounts, to supplement the vitamins you receive in your food."

Linus Pauling
(Winner of 2 Nobel Prizes, 1901-1994)

The YFH HealthPrint

Initially, our services were only available through physicians or by referral. The early YFH program was effective, but somewhat expensive because we worked personally with a small client base on a one-to-one basis.

But the health benefits of our customized results were so impressive that it was always our objective to somehow bring our costs down and make the program affordable to everyone. It took a number of years to work out the details, but we finally began offering the YFH HealthPrint nationally in 1999. Now, anyone wishing to take direct control of his or her health can do so with the HealthPrint self-help program. It isn't necessary to go through your doctor to get a HealthPrint. However, YFH does suggest that you provide your doctor with your laboratory test results.

A HealthPrint is a complete package that includes fifty-seven of the most essential blood tests processed at our state-of-the-art reference lab. The test results are tabulated in an easy-to-understand manner, and an extensive interpretive guide is customized for you. The Guide explains what each result means, and how to raise, lower, or maintain your current levels in the optimum range for each test. It also includes a toll-free help line for questions you may have.

I believe a HealthPrint is the most complete and accurate set of preventive blood tests available. In addition, our Interpretive Guide (over 200 pages of recommendations for using your blood test results most effectively) is a comprehensive resource that recommends dietary and lifestyle changes based on lab results.

So how does it work?

The first step in the HealthPrint program is for you to have your blood drawn at one of thousands of participating collection sites with which we are associated throughout the country. The draw takes less than five minutes, does not require a doctor's appointment, and the cost is included in the HealthPrint package.

YFH then does a comprehensive series of tests on your blood sample. Most of the tests are listed in Part III of this book. Because we're a large processor, our lab costs are lower than the prices our clients or their physicians would be offered, and we pass these savings on to you.

Beyond the tests included in the basic HealthPrint, we also offer specialized tests that clients with particular needs may wish to add. We offer specific tests that are highly predictive for cancer. We offer extensive heart packages, and several special tests that are hard to find and are especially valuable if repeated and tracked over time. One such test is the Omega 3 Profile+.

After your blood draw, you receive your results for the fifty-seven parameters in the mail, along with the Interpretive Guide. The YFH HealthPrint Guide suggests extensive diet and lifestyle recommendations to improve or maintain your results based on your own unique biochemistry. These recommendations are made without conflict of interest, since YFH does not sell nutritional supplements or any other nutritional product.

Preventive blood testing and nutritional interpretation of the results is YFH's specialty. Feel free to contact YFH if you need help knowing which tests would be most beneficial for you.

Visit our Web site:

www.yourfuturehealth.com

Or

Call our toll-free telephone number:

1-877-GO TO YFH
1-877-468-6934

Our address:

Your Future Health
P.O. Box 1369
Tavares, Florida 32778

Family and friends have encouraged me to develop a book on heart disease, exploring both its relationship to other degenerative diseases, and long-term prevention and treatment. While working on that project, I decided to add a new chapter that follows to provide an early look at this exciting new material, "Heart Disease – No More!"

"All we need to make us really happy is something to be enthusiastic about."

Albert Einstein
(1921 Nobel Prize Winner, 1879-1955)

Heart Disease - No More!

Fifty years ago heart disease was responsible for more deaths in the US than any other disease. The sad fact is that despite our many technological advances in the last half century, the statistics haven't changed.

A major reason that heart disease continues to be the number one killer in the US and around the world is that we still don't fully understand all the nuances of this disease. Each time we improve our knowledge of its causes, a single treatment solution emerges—promoted as—*the* answer to ending heart disease once and for all. Among these single factors, researchers have pointed to plaque buildup, inflammation, supplement deficiencies or excesses, AA/EPA ratios, total cholesterol, homocysteine, or C-reactive protein levels.

A single isolated solution, however, is unlikely to be the answer to any complex disease. What is really needed is a comprehensive approach. Many avenues of early detection are available and should all be used. These include a physical exam, extensive blood testing, and in many cases, additional specialty tests. A health improvement program is optimally effective when *all* these modalities are used. A successful program starts with blood testing and goes on to include nutrition, stress management, exercise and understanding blood tests genetics.

Since my area of expertise is customized nutritional interpretations of blood tests, this chapter focuses on the blood tests required to detect heart disease at its earliest stages. It also describes how to establish a meaningful trend based on blood test results, plus a brief summary of what heart disease is and why it is called the "silent killer."

What is Heart Disease?

Heart disease is defined as a set of conditions that lead to heart attack, stroke, or cardiac arrest. Heart attacks occur when the blood supply to part of the heart is severely curtailed or blocked. Typically, a heart attack occurs when plaque forms in an artery, blocking blood supply to the heart. Plaque formation can lead to clot formation, especially if the blood is thick and/or sticky. An excess of red blood cells and/or platelets can make the blood thick and the blood can be sticky when there is an overabundance of glucose. A clot can form and eventually break loose and lodge in a narrowed or partially blocked area of a blood vessel causing blood flow to slow down or stop.

Strokes occur when blood vessels to the brain are blocked by clots or when they burst (often due to high blood pressure). When this happens, the brain cannot get blood or oxygen, so it begins to die. Sometimes people experience what is called a "mini-stroke." Mini-strokes occur when the brain is still able to get some blood and oxygen, but not enough, causing confusion and lack of mental acuity. This is a more frequent occurrence than most people realize because mini-strokes often appear totally undetected. Mini-strokes may emerge when smaller blood vessels burst; or, when red blood cells that carry oxygen to the brain are not healthy or are not produced in sufficient quantity, reducing the oxygen supply.

Cardiac arrest occurs when there is an abrupt loss of heart function. Typically, the coronary arteries are narrowed by fatty buildups. Fatty buildups attract bacteria. Bacteria can form when the blood is "sweet," that is, when glucose levels are higher than normal, providing food for the bacteria. The excess bacteria causes an increase in white blood cells (white blood cells kill bacteria). If the immune system is not strong enough to protect against the bacteria, inflammation develops. Inflammation can actually cause the heart to stop. This is how heart disease, Diabetes (excess sugar) and inflammation are connected.

Sweet dessert → fatty buildup → increased blood glucose → bacteria → gathering of white blood cells → weakened immune system → inflammation → may lead to serious disease, including cardiac arrest

---

Why is heart disease known as the "silent killer"?

Heart disease is known as the silent killer because significant damage takes place while the victim is totally unaware that anything so health-destructive is going on. Almost all of us know people who "suddenly" dropped dead because of a heart attack, even though that person appeared to be the picture of health. These people looked good and felt good. Many people live with severely blocked and/or inflamed blood vessels for years before developing overt symptoms of heart disease. We have seen clients who had 95 percent blockages before they experienced their first symptom. (Sadly, this was usually a heart attack.) The point is "feeling good" isn't good enough.

This is why accurate cardiovascular blood testing is a necessity and why assuming that you are healthy because your score is within the reference range is not correct. It is imperative that heart disease be detected early so that relatively simple corrective measures can be put in place. If you wait for heart disease symptoms, the range of corrective alternatives is greatly reduced and the options that are left, such as drugs or surgery, have serious side effects and risks.

Which blood tests need to be done as part of a comprehensive heart disease prevention program?

The necessary tests:
- Basic HealthPrint (complete chemistry panel that includes 57 measures including a manual differential as well as Zinc and Magnesium)

- Omega 3 Profile+ (Includes Omega 3 Score and Serum Phospholipid AA/EPA Ratio, plus other omega 3 and omega 6 fatty acids)
- Homocysteine
- C-Reactive Protein
- Ferritin
- VAP (genetic cholesterol test)
- Fasting Insulin
- A-1-C Hemoglobin
- Thyroid Panel
- Progesterone

Detailed information about each of these tests is included in the "Essential Blood Test Reference Guide" in Part III.

As stated earlier, it is imperative that all tests be repeated and the results tracked and compared. At the very least the Basic HealthPrint, Omega 3 Profile+, Homocysteine, C-Reactive Protein & Ferritin tests should be repeated yearly. One of the greatest benefits of annual testing is that it allows for comparison, helping to spot trend irregularities early on. To ensure optimum health, each of the cancer screens should also be done yearly. Be sure to read the Case Study section that follows this chapter to learn how many YFH clients – with a wide variety of health challenges – have benefited from following this advice.

As discussed in "All Blood Tests are Not Created Equal," to produce valid results for comparison, the correct protocol *must* be followed. *Even using the same lab may not ensure accuracy because the lab analyzes what it receives most often without knowledge of how the sample was treated or the collection protocol that was followed before its arrival. This could make a big difference for the accuracy of the result.*

The collection process and preparation for shipping as well as analysis methods must be consistent. Recommendations to take corrective action towards optimum health depend on getting the baseline score, retesting at least yearly with the same methodology, and recording these valid results over time.

Why are the recommended blood tests important to a comprehensive understanding of heart disease, and how can they help the implementation of corrective action in a timely fashion?

Test	Issues Test Will Uncover	Interpretations Will Help
Basic HealthPrint	Helps identify sticky blood, thick blood, inflammation, blood density, various chemical imbalances, hormone levels, immune system deficiencies, bacteria, viruses	Improve oxidation of cells, improve circulation, strengthen immune system, balance systems (electrolytes, protein, minerals), improve kidney and liver health, thereby cleansing the blood
Omega 3 Profile +	Risk for heart disease, inflammation, immune system deficiencies, weight loss challenges	Increase level of Omega 3' s, improve circulation, strengthen immune system, improve mental acuity and reduce depression

table continued on next page

VAP	Genetic risk of heart disease, specific cholesterol (lipoprotein) density subset levels, triglyceride level	Improve specific cholesterol (lipoprotein) density and triglyceride levels; manage the effect of genetic heart issues
Homocysteine	Specific protein amino acid level	Balance essential amino acid methionine metabolism, thereby reducing tendency for blood cells to stick
C-Reactive Protein	Bacteria and/or virus presence	Reduce infection/inflammation
Ferritin	Iron utilization inside cells	Reduce inflammation (excess iron attracts bacteria, which can cause inflammation), increase oxygenation of cells

As a result of my extensive experience, I have concluded that all ten tests detailed in these two tables should be done as a baseline and repeated yearly. I realize how expensive it is to do all ten tests annually. The first six tests (see first table) are essential, with the exception of the VAP. One would do the VAP at least yearly if the cholesterol density pattern is an A/B or B. However, if the pattern is A, then you may wish to do the VAP every two years. If finances are not an issue, the VAP and the additional four tests (see following table) should also be done every year.

Fasting Insulin	Insulin level imbalances	Balance arachidonic acid and glucose, thereby reducing tendency for blood to stick, improve circulation, provide a way to measure the effects of stress
A-1-C Hemoglobin	Glucose level imbalances	Balance insulin/glucose levels, thereby reducing tendency towards sweet, sticky blood and reducing tendency for bacteria to feed on it, improving circulation, and reducing inflammation
Custom Thyroid Panel and Free T4	Metabolism issues and hormone imbalance	Improve metabolism and sleep patterns, balance heart beat and pulse levels, control weight, reduce depression, reduce menopause/cardiac symptoms
Progesterone	Progesterone and estrogen imbalance	Balancing progesterone and estrogen can improve heart rate, reduce menopause/cardiac symptoms, and improve weight control and libido

For more information about symptoms and their relationship to specific tests, please see Part IV.

Why are so many tests recommended?

Heart disease can be the result of a combination of many factors. Some of these include: stress, sticky blood, blood cholesterol density, inherited genetic anomalies, bacteria or viruses present in the blood, glucose irregularities, abnormal insulin levels, vessel constrictions due to plaque buildup, inflammation, levels of various chemicals (such as caffeine), and amino acid imbalances. Clearly, a simple Total Cholesterol test is not the solution to the early discovery of heart disease.

What are the various factors that play a role in heart disease, and what tests can be done to detect them early enough to facilitate corrections before serious damage is done?

Factors	Symptoms	Tests
Sticky blood	Blood sugar (glucose) too high, clots form	A-1-C Hemoglobin, VAP, Fasting Insulin, Omega 3 Profile +, HealthPrint (includes Fasting Glucose)
Sticky blood (continued)	Excess homocysteine, (Amino Acid imbalance) clots form, plaque deposits	Homocysteine, Omega 3 Profile +, VAP, HealthPrint
Sticky blood (continued)	Excess triglycerides, plaque deposits, clots form	VAP, Omega 3 Profile +, HealthPrint (Includes Fasting Glucose)
Thick Blood	Excess red or white blood cells or platelets, clots form	Omega 3 Profile +, HealthPrint (includes complete blood count with manual red cell morphology and white blood cell differential)

table continued on next page

Blood Vessel Restrictions	Plaque formation on interior of blood vessel walls causes narrowing of blood vessel and rough surface for blood cells to stick to and clot, high blood pressure due to small opening for blood flow, also causing weakened blood vessels to burst	VAP, Omega 3 Profile +, Custom Thyroid Panel, Free T4, HealthPrint
Genetic Factors	Cholesterol density pattern high risk, more likely to form plaque, blood more apt to stick to vessels forming plaque	VAP, Omega 3 Profile +
Stress	Constriction of arteries and/or veins may even reduce blood flow to/from cells, immune system can be weakened and oxygen carrying capacity can be reduced, and nutrient deficiencies can contribute to all of these issues	Omega 3 Profile +, HealthPrint (includes manual RBC morphology, CBC and WBC differential as well as tests to identify nutritional deficiencies), Ferritin, Custom Thyroid Panel, Free T4
Various Chemical and/or Hormone Level Imbalances	Major organs not properly supporting the heart and cardiovascular system	Omega 3 Profile +, HealthPrint (includes fasting glucose, 5 Liver and 4 Kidney tests), Custom Thyroid Panel, Free T4, Progesterone

In addition to controlling heart disease, will these suggestions help with other health problems?

The steps recommended in this chapter not only help keep heart disease at bay, but can also help control diabetes, cancer, excess weight and degenerative diseases of all kinds. All of these health challenges are caused by poor oxygenation of cells, poor nutrient absorption, and/ or poor delivery of nutrients to the cells, as well as inefficient removal of waste from cells due to lack of exercise and improper electrolyte balance.

The protocol is easy to recommend, but not so easy to follow. I myself struggle to consistently abide by this system even though I know that it works when I do. We can only succeed from the efforts of our hard work. No one can do it for us. Just take it one day at a time. If you falter, start again and try not to get angry with yourself. Your body won't give up on you if you don't give up on it.

In Conclusion

Although this chapter (I am told) is power packed and may seem overwhelming at times, I want to encourage you to read and reread it and share it with others you love. The material I have presented may be the most important words contained in this book because heart disease affects us all either directly or indirectly.

In fact, most of my immediate family members have the worst possible genetic cholesterol density pattern for cardiovascular and related diseases. Our family medical history is riddled with heart disease as well as diabetes and six different types of cancer. This is one of the reasons that I am so passionate about developing a dependable detection system which, when used regularly, helps protect against these debilitating diseases.

In summary, I feel the need to reiterate that heart disease remains the number one killer as of this writing not because we do not have the knowledge or technology to control it, but because we do not understand how to use the knowledge and technology we already possess for early detection. Now that you know what action is needed, I hope you will make a commitment to test at least yearly and make Heart Disease—No More!

Now I would like to encourage you to take a look at Part II, the Case Study section. You will meet a number of people who have worked with YFH to solve specific health problems.

Case Studies on Blood Testing,

Nutrition and Specific Diseases

This section focuses on the benefits offered by nutritionally interpreted blood testing for the alleviation and/or management of specific illnesses and disease.

It is beyond the scope of this book to cover everything about blood testing, cancer, heart disease or any other single medical condition. But I believe we can discuss the most important points.

To accomplish that goal, I'd like to introduce a few of the clients with whom we've worked. Their situations are, for the most part, quite common in Western society. However, what worked for them would not necessarily be applicable to others facing similar health problems. Again, I must stress that even if symptoms, age, gender, height and weight, etc., are the same, the solution for each individual would most likely be very different. Therefore, please do not assume that what worked for the people you are going to read about will work for you.

Heart Disease & Diabetes

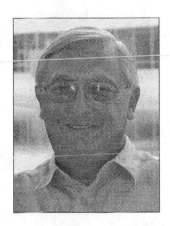

Background
Dr. Jeffrey Kramer is a retired optometrist who practiced in New York, and currently lives in Florida.

The Problem
When we began working with Dr. Kramer about sixteen years ago, he was overweight, diabetic, and like all diabetics, had blood circulation and cardiovascular problems. He was already taking the maximum possible oral dose of insulin-regulating drugs, and had just been told by his doctor, a leading endocrinologist, that he needed to start insulin injections. He knew that long-term insulin injections could have negative health effects. He began working with YFH as part of his search for an alternative solution.

His YFH Blood Tests
Dr. Kramer's blood sugar level of 188, even while on insulin-regulating medication, was very high. (Optimum is around 90-100.) His cholesterol was also high at 325, and his HDL to overall cholesterol ratio was an astounding 14.8. (Below 2.5 is optimum.) His triglycerides were a whopping 1430 (a score of 50 is good). These scores had been seriously abnormal for at least a decade.

What We Recommended

We recommended a dramatic diet change that eliminated virtually all carbohydrates. He shifted his attention to eating more animal proteins, nuts, and low carbohydrate and low glycemic (low insulin-producing) vegetables. In addition, we suggested a protein supplement and a relatively large daily dose of B-complex vitamins, lecithin, vitamins C and E, chromium, zinc, EPA, DHA and GLA to nourish his pancreas and regulate insulin production. We also encouraged him to drink as much water as possible. A diet so high in protein required careful kidney monitoring, so he did a complete HealthPrint with YFH every four months. He also tested his blood sugar and cholesterol with his doctor each month.

His Results

Over time, Jeff's triglycerides dropped to a reasonable 196, and his overall cholesterol went down to 163 without the use of any cholesterol-lowering drugs.

After more than a decade of chronically bad blood chemistry, we found it difficult to get most of his scores into YFH optimum ranges. But we were gratified for what we were able to accomplish, since his level of blood vessel plaque could have led to a stroke, dangerously high blood pressure, or a heart attack. Instead, he lowered his weight, increased his energy level, and improved his circulation, which enabled him to pass all his stress tests.

After years of elevated scores, his internist felt that a routine Doppler study (ultrasound) was indicated. This showed that his primary arteries leading to his heart were

95 percent blocked. His cardiologist thought a quadruple bypass would be necessary.

His doctors were mystified, since other than the results of the Doppler study, he appeared to be getting adequate blood circulation to his heart. This suggested the need for further tests, and an MRI revealed something extraordinary. He had grown new blood vessels around each blocked blood vessel. We were all astounded and gratified.

Needless to say, Jeff did not need a quadruple bypass after all. By following YFH dietary recommendations, he was able to get his blood sugar under control, eliminate the need to take insulin injections, or even continue his oral medications. His health is now excellent, and he's actively enjoying a well-deserved retirement.

General Conclusions

Growing new blood vessels around a blockage demonstrates what the body can do to heal itself when nutrition is optimized to the body's unique biochemical needs. Recent US and Italian research studies confirm that the human heart can generate new blood vessels. Dr. Kramer was absolutely determined not to go on insulin, so he never cheated on his diet, and followed all YFH recommendations. He was responsible for his success. His internist managed his medications and offered support. YFH acted as the coach, a practice we extend to all our HealthPrint clients.

While his focus was primarily to avoid insulin by working to balance his blood chemistry, he achieved improvements in all of his biological systems—most dramatically, in his cardiovascular health.

What is especially interesting about him is that he achieved these extraordinary health gains by improving his blood scores, but without getting many of them into YFH optimum ranges. He is a classic example of a client whose Personal Normal scores were not optimum for his height, weight, age and gender but were so drastically improved that his body responded nonetheless. After years of not making the right diet and lifestyle choices, he could not immediately optimize his blood chemistry. However, he achieved impressive improvements, suggesting that it is never too late to start living in a more healthful manner.

Conclusions about Heart Disease

There's no mystery as to how we develop heart disease, the number one killer in the US today. The primary cause? Unhealthful diet and lifestyle choices—with their concomitant chronically bad blood chemistry.

We often see blood scores that indicate impending cardiovascular disease. This is tragic. We know heart disease isn't necessary, nor is it inevitable even if your parents had it. And, as Jeff exemplifies, it's never too late to turn things around. Rereading "Heart Disease—No More!" provides more details.

Conclusions about Diabetes

Like heart disease, adult onset diabetes can be prevented in a large number of cases. One out of every two Americans has low blood sugar (hypoglycemia) and doesn't know it. The condition goes unnoticed and unchecked. Low blood sugar results in an overproduction of insulin. After years of overproducing insulin, the pancreas becomes erratic in its production and then almost stops insulin production completely causing the blood sugar to rise above normal. This condition is referred to as hyperglycemia or diabetes.

As blood sugar levels continue to rise over the years, people are told that they are normal—until their blood sugar level climbs high enough to be diagnosed with adult onset diabetes. The vast majority of people who have this disease once had undiagnosed hypoglycemia (overproduction of insulin). Recognizing hypoglycemia in the earliest stage provides the time to make serious changes to one's diet and lifestyle—changes usually allow the pancreas to balance its production of insulin.

Maintaining an optimum blood sugar level through diet, and keeping track of blood glucose levels through blood testing, can avert the development of adult onset diabetes.

Cancer

Background

Ray Miller (photo next page) had always enjoyed robust good health without working at it too hard. He lives in a small town in Ohio, and works as a salesman.

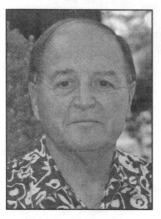

The Problem

Several years ago, Ray developed a sharp pain in the back of his neck that wouldn't go away. His doctor hospitalized him for testing, and he was diagnosed with lymphoma of the neck near the cervical spine, and a soft tissue mass on the pancreas that was malignant. Cancer.

Ray began radiation therapy immediately. The radiation was not successful—no tumor shrinkage, no improvement of condition, the cancer was metastasizing (spreading) so his doctors put him on chemotherapy and told him his condition was probably terminal. They suggested that he get his affairs in order. YFH started working with him just as he was beginning chemotherapy.

His YFH Blood Tests

Ray's blood chemistry was in poor shape. His red blood cell count (RBC) was very low, and his cells were abnormally shaped. His hemoglobin was also very low (it was around 11). Relative to his YFH optimum ranges, his hematocrit, zinc, white blood cell count, blood sugar, protein, calcium and magnesium were all low. The low scores were partially due to the chemotherapy, but in looking at his old records, we discovered that he'd had low red blood cell counts for quite some time, as do most people who develop cancer. His blood analysis suggested poor circulation and poor oxygenation of tissue—that is, poor ability to get proper oxygen supply to his cells. When this occurs for an extended period of time, cancer can develop.

What We Recommended

Ray's HealthPrint suggested a complete diet and lifestyle change. He ate organic meats, poultry, fish, nuts, organic whole grain breads and lots of organic, low carbohydrate, low glycemic vegetables. He chose not to consume alcohol or caffeine, and instead used high doses of B complex, E, A, C, chromium, zinc, and essential fatty acid supplements. We suggested that he take time every day to relax, use laughter therapy, exercise, and be upbeat and positive.

The chemotherapy had taken away his strength, but Ray fought to do what he could. He told us about a small hill behind his house that was covered with trees. At the beginning he was too weak to even walk up the hill, but as often as he could, he crawled up the hill just to sit, commune with nature, and meditate. He, his family and his friends also filled his life with prayer. He was determined to overcome his cancer, no matter what it took.

Ray reported that his doctors weren't in favor of the nutrition plan he was following. But Ray insisted on following it anyway, because he felt that most traditional doctors were out of their area of expertise when advising about nutrition.

His Results

Six months after beginning the YFH program, Ray was in remission. His doctor told him that his cancer was gone.

The doctor didn't know how it disappeared, but clearly it was gone. When he heard the news, he went to the parking lot and cried tears of joy.

That was almost eight years ago, and Ray is still in remission. His strength is back, he's working again, and he tells us that the only change from his previous life is that he no longer has any bad days. Every day is a great day and he's a lot more emotional than he used to be.

General Conclusions

Cancer involving the pancreas is almost always fatal. Ray credits his cure to traditional and complementary/alternative therapies, and spiritual approaches working together, as well as his steely determination to overcome his illness.

Chemotherapy and radiation kill cancer cells, but they also kill healthy tissue. YFH worked to restore Ray's immune system strength after it had broken down from cancer and chemotherapy.

Doctors sometimes tell their patients, as did Ray's doctor, that they shouldn't do any sort of special nutrition or supplement program during chemotherapy. It is true that some chemotherapy drugs are rendered ineffective if certain vitamins are taken at the time of treatment. The question to ask is what food needs to be avoided? Good supplements for cancer patients are usually made from food and rarely interfere with chemotherapy. However, depending on the drug, YFH suggests not using any supplements that may block a drug's effectiveness the day of and day after the treatment.

While a "one-size-fits-all" nutrition program might not be helpful, a customized nutrition plan developed for you from an analysis of your blood can restore balance to your blood chemistry—balance that has been lost due to radiation and chemotherapy treatments. In my clinical work over the decades, I've seen that customized nutrition is essential during a time when your body is being broken down both by the disease and, temporarily, by the treatment.

Now let's review another case study where the client had pancreatic cancer but without needing chemotherapy and radiation. We just discussed Ray who used our system for blood testing and nutritional interventions after he discovered his cancer and after traditional treatment. Unlike Ray, Judy found her cancer in time to avoid chemotherapy and radiation and used blood testing preventively. Our preventive early detection system helped Judy find the disease at its earliest stage.

Pancreatic Disease

Background
Judy (photo next page) has been a nurse for over 40 years, which includes hospice care for 12 of those years. She is over 60 and regularly plays on a traveling tennis team. She decided to become a nurse to help others. Recently, this decision helped save her life. She was always motivated to find a way to take a proactive approach to

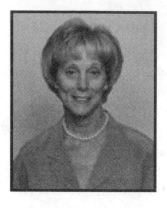

her health. She had medical concerns that were not getting better with normal intervention. A colleague suggested testing with YFH.

Judy credits YFH with saving her from dying from pancreatic cancer. Survival was unlikely if she had not utilized preventive blood testing.

The Problem

Judy's *original problem* was hypertension or high blood pressure and like Katherine Hepburn, her head would shake uncontrollably at times. She also had heart arrhythmia attacks and her usual high energy level was lacking. According to our nutritional interpretation, she had the following deficiencies: potassium, magnesium, vitamins A, B-complex, additional vitamin B6, C, E, zinc and lecithin. Her symptoms have been controlled by continuing her medication and adding our nutrient suggestions. Testing her blood to find the correct balance of supplementation and diet changes and then implementing the changes produced a quick turn-around for her. She was pleased with her results and has continued to test preventively with YFH since January of 1997.

The problem that developed next left Judy speechless. We found reason to suspect precancerous pancreatic disease, one of the most deadly cancers. YFH had consistently suggested that perhaps her job was too stressful. We encouraged her to change nursing specialties or to be more committed to a stress management program. Regular exercise was not enough to reduce her stress.

There were signs in her blood that showed less than optimum ability to oxygenate, nourish, cleanse and defend her cells from disease. She had nine scores that were lower than usual and four scores that were higher than usual (for Judy). Because these scores were not outside the normal reference range, she did not feel the need to make meaningful changes to her lifestyle.

Since this less than optimum trend continued, in late 2001, YFH encouraged her to have a CEA test. (A carcinocmbiyonic antigen test which is usually done to measure the effectiveness of someone undergoing chemotherapy or when specific cancers are strongly suspected. Her symptoms would not have justified ordering this test normally). However, YFH has found that the CEA test can be very useful in the early discovery of many cancers in their precancerous state.

Our empirical research on the CEA test has been most powerful. Five years ago we began tracking CEA data in combination with our HealthPrint program and additional test history provided by patients' doctors. When accurately analyzed, this test—compared with previous results—can actually find certain cancers early on. Cancers such as lung, pancreatic, liver, bone, breast, thyroid, and intestinal cancers from the stomach to the colon. Now YFH encourages every client to have this test done yearly to establish scores for comparison.

Her YFH Blood Tests

Judy took our advice and added the CEA to her usual test regimen. Much to our chagrin, her first score of 3.1 was above the normal reference range of 2.6. We like to see scores below 1.0 for everyone, but naturally some people (like me for example) have scores higher than 2.6 and yet this is still normal. We encouraged her to call her doctor and have a retest done in one month just to be sure the score did not continue to rise.

Because her first test was abnormal, subsequent tests if ordered by her doctor would be covered by insurance. Her doctor did not feel that the score was too alarming but to be on the safe side he ran the test in three months and found that it was even higher. He then retested the CEA again three months later and found the score rose even higher to 4.2. At this point, he decided to send Judy to an oncologist for a second opinion.

As can happen sometimes, the oncologist did not feel that a score of 3.1, jumping to 4.2 was significant because in his world, patients have scores of 200 when he first tests them. He told Judy that she had no reason to be alarmed and that in fact she had wasted her money all these years testing with YFH. Today we find more and more doctors aligning with our preventive blood test methodology. We thank our medical advisory board members and participating doctors for helping us to change this way of thinking.

Fortunately for Judy, her personal doctor referred her to another oncologist who ran the additional tests needed and found precancerous pancreatic cancer (pancreatic cancer in its infancy stage). Needless to say this was her greatest fear, but we felt confident that the outcome would be positive because the disease was discovered so early.

This is a good time to pause and reflect. How could Judy develop such a deadly cancer when she tested regularly and tried to follow our principles? We must remember that stress is our greatest enemy. While the purpose of testing is to stay healthy, sometimes we cannot overcome the effect of life's stresses. Therefore, the best we can do is find disease early enough to remove it before it spreads and causes irreversible damage. In most cases, we no longer need to fear discovering that we have cancer or other diseases. What we must fear is not finding it in time.

Judy did just that, and had a modified Whipple surgical procedure to remove her tumor. Her tumor was still sitting on the outside of the pancreas wall without invading it or spreading to any surrounding organs. She was able to keep her pancreas and return to her normal duties within a few weeks.

What We Recommended
We stepped up our nutritional suggestions for Judy as soon as we received the first CEA test score of 3.1 in an effort to protect her during the discovery phase, just in case she had cancer. Some of the changes included the addition of EPA, GLA, more zinc, acidophilus, L lysine, and more of the vitamins that are destroyed by stress, such as vitamins A, E, B complex, and C. We suggested

that she improve her diet and eat only the best quality of whole foods. We strongly advised no cheating, which Judy, like so many of us, is guilty of from time to time. Naturally, we also suggested more frequent checkups for the CEA, and that she continued getting HealthPrints for the rest of her life. Now she tests every six months without fail. (If the CEA or any other test takes a sudden jump, she will test as often as needed until her scores return to her personal normal.)

Her Results

Judy has tested several times with YFH since her surgery. We are thrilled to report that her CEA scores are steady at 3.1 every time. Her HealthPrint scores are improving as well. Her zinc, direct bilirubin and total bilirubin look good, uric acid better than ever, and her red blood cell distribution is also back to normal, including the number of red blood cells and their size, shape, and color. We have some work to do to correct her Omega 3 Profile+ test for arachidonic acid and her glucose scores, but she is well on her way to optimum health once again. She is back to playing tennis and she says she feels great. Her new passion is to help others understand the devastating effect of stress on health. In fact, she is writing a book that is sure to be loved by all who read it.

We expect it will be some time before her CEA scores go down below 3.1, but we are all happy that it is so much lower than 4.2 she experienced only a few months ago. She has been given a clean bill of health by her regular doctor who stood by her from the beginning. Judy and her husband Roger could not be happier with the outcome. Their greatest hope is that their willingness to share her story will perhaps help you or someone you know some day.

General Conclusions

Judy said it best in an interview with Fox and CBS news when she said, "I hope everyone who hears my story will be called to action. I feel strongly that everyone would benefit from preventive blood testing. If you wait until you have symptoms, it is often too late. I found a tumor from one of the deadliest cancers before any symptoms appeared and for that I thank YFH."

Obesity

Background

Sharon Murphy lives in an urban area of Ohio, and has been doing preventive blood testing with YFH for more than fifteen years.

What's unique about Sharon is that until recently, she did YFH blood tests at least once a year. Sharon never followed our suggestions for diet or lifestyle changes. She continued to eat lots of cookies, candy and soft drinks, and didn't let the extra forty pounds she carried bother her too much. She would have liked to lower her weight, but felt that it would be impossible for her. She told us she'd make changes to improve her health if and when her blood chemistry ever started to deteriorate. And for years she got away with it.

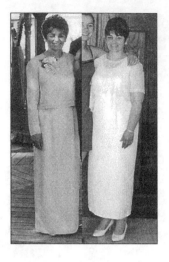

The Problem

Eventually, Sharon's blood scores began to worsen. She developed pain in her legs and started to sense a decline in mental acuity. Around this time, she went to her nephew's wedding. After seeing the wedding photos, she felt she "looked like a hippopotamus." Her daughter was to be married the following year, and she resolved then and there that as the mother of the bride, she was not going to be overweight for *that* wedding.

Her father had also recently passed away. He'd always been healthy, but a cardiovascular condition had come on fast, and he'd rapidly gone down hill. It seemed to her that messages were coming at her from all directions. It was time to finally improve her diet and lifestyle. She called YFH and asked for help developing a detailed plan that would improve her health and help her lose the excess pounds.

Her YFH Blood Tests

Sharon's main problems were low blood sugar, which suggested pending adult onset diabetes, and higher than optimum cholesterol. Her thyroid function was also sub-optimum although still normal. As noted in the case of Dr. Kramer, diabetes and heart disease go hand in hand, and the writing was on the wall for what she would be facing if she didn't improve her diet and lifestyle.

What We Recommended

Sharon's HealthPrint recommended a diet rich in proteins, plus low carbohydrate, low glycemic vegetables. She eliminated all the junk food carbohydrates along with caffeine from her diet. She doesn't like fruit, so she took concentrated fruit and vegetable powder capsules. She took supplements like seaweed, as well as EPA fish oil (to nourish her thyroid), B complex, potassium, vitamin C, and a general multiple vitamin. She had a protein shake for breakfast every day. She simply ate the right foods for her own biology and never counted calories. She took an equally informal approach to working out—a brisk walk every day, no elaborate workout programs.

Her Results

It took Sharon about seven months to lose 35 pounds, and another 5 months to lose the remaining five pounds. By the time her daughter's wedding day arrived, she'd reached her goal of being 40 pounds lighter. The pictures of her (photos previous page) were taken pre and post weight loss. The one on the right was taken at her nephew's wedding when she weighed over 150 pounds. The one on the left was taken at her daughter's wedding, where she weighed 114. She's kept the weight off for the past two years, and by following the right diet, she has even lost a few additional pounds.

In addition to losing weight, she succeeded in maximizing her health. She normalized her blood sugar, optimized her thyroid function, lowered her cholesterol, and improved her general metabolism—burning calories the way she should. This made it easy to keep her weight constant. She no longer had any pain in her legs, and slept better at night. She even felt her mental acuity sharpen.

General Conclusions

For some people an unhealthful diet and lifestyle contribute to a serious decline in health. In one sense, these are the lucky ones, because they can easily listen to their bodies and know just how far they can go without risking their health. But for many, health appears to be robust enough to survive neglect for years, without palpable symptoms. This is a shame because lifestyle will eventually take its toll whether you "feel" the warnings or not.

In Sharon's case, her blood chemistry did not worsen after many years of neglect, even though she was overweight—until her forty-eighth year. If her health problems were not addressed, they could have led to heart disease and diabetes.

If you care mainly about losing weight, a customized diet developed for your own blood chemistry is a super way of cutting pounds naturally, without risk. Why does it work? Because it's developed from and for your own metabolism, and that makes all the difference. Anyone can design a weight-loss diet, but it may not make you healthier. It is best to test your blood before starting any weight loss program and to test again when you complete the regimen.

Infertility and Miscarriage

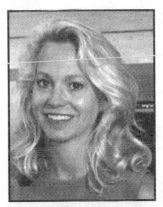

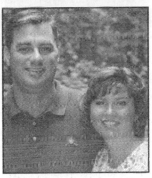

Background and Problem

Becky Distad-Rossi (top photo) has a five-year-old son, but she and her husband had been unable to conceive a second child.

Scott and Bridget (bottom photo) had been attempting to conceive for over six years without success.

Ron and Kristin DiNardo (photo next page) were able to conceive, but Kristin was unable to carry to term. Her first three pregnancies had resulted in miscarriages.

All three couples had been to fertility clinics, and had spent thousands of dollars on procedures that had not been successful. They all had begun to despair that their plans for children—or for additional children—would not be possible.

What they all found frustrating was that the specialists at the fertility clinics were unable to adequately explain why they weren't able to conceive or carry to term. Becky had been told that she might be too old at age thirty-eight. Kristin had been told that she might be allergic to her husband. Scott and Bridget were told nothing at all.

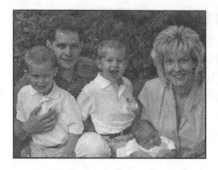

All began working with YFH after exhausting other options.

Their YFH Blood Analyses

YFH ran comprehensive blood tests on Becky (her husband tested later), Bridget, Scott, Kristin and Ron. The most striking deficiency in all five cases was zinc. The three women all had under-performing thyroid function. In all five cases, blood glucose, hemoglobin, red blood cell counts, magnesium, progesterone and essential fatty acids were normal but not optimum.

What We Recommended

YFH has seen in the past that zinc deficiency, especially when coupled with less than optimum thyroid and other blood chemistry factors, could result in dramatically reduced fertility or ability to carry a pregnancy to term. Zinc plays such a large role in pregnancy because it works to stimulate and regulate most hormone activity in the body. (Zinc and magnesium, by the way, were the two major blood chemistry parameters that had never been checked by any of the five at the fertility clinics.)

Each couple optimized their diet and supplements, based on their blood panel results. They corrected thyroid function imbalances and built up zinc levels.

Their Results

Within a few months after starting the YFH program, Becky became pregnant, and had a healthy son.

Scott and Bridget also conceived in short order, and gave birth to a healthy son, Timothy.

Kristin became pregnant within three months, carried the pregnancy to term, and gave birth to a healthy son. She has since given birth two other healthy children. She has not had another miscarriage, since beginning the YFH program.

All three couples were not using fertility drugs before or during these pregnancies. All three feel that they would not have been able to realize their plans for children without the YFH nutritional program, which was, as always, customized to their own unique biochemistries.

General Conclusions

Within the next few years, I suspect that zinc may begin to be considered something of a miracle supplement. For the moment, serum zinc deficiencies tend to be overlooked in medical diagnosis. As a result, a number of afflictions that would be easily treated with zinc supplementation go untreated and unresolved.

Why is this? Because zinc is hard to test accurately! Serum zinc levels must be prepared for analysis almost immediately after a blood draw. Most collection sites send their blood samples out for this preparation and analysis, and proper zinc sample preparation is delayed. This skews the results. Few labs currently offer zinc testing in-house. Since zinc evaluations are hard to come by, they are rarely ordered. It's also difficult to build up the right serum zinc level without regular blood testing—too much zinc can be as bad as too little. It's well worth the effort to get serum nutritional zinc levels optimized. In addition to the area of fertility, many of our clients have improved or corrected long-standing medical problems largely as a result of correcting serum zinc deficiencies.

Balancing <u>all</u> the blood chemistry parameters tends to repair whatever is wrong. This is why YFH does so many tests—between fifty-seven and seventy separate blood tests for each client. To optimize all of your body's biological systems, you need to know how each body system utilizes nutrients individually and collectively.

Digestion

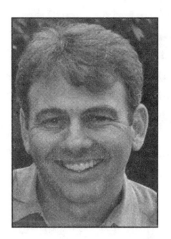

Background and Problem

Tim Muldoon is a businessman. Dr. Richard Krantz (photo next page) is a dentist. Both have been plagued by irritable bowel syndrome all their lives. Tim had a chronically over-active bowel, gas and cramps. Richard had a chronically under-active bowel and constipation. As a result, both dreaded the prospect of eating. Each had been to numerous specialists, and each had

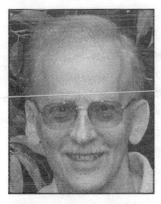

been told that no cure was available for his respective condition. Learn to live with it, the doctors said.

Their YFH Blood Tests

Both had extremely low levels of magnesium. The deficiency was much worse for Richard. Tim's thyroid was under-active. Both had zinc deficiencies—again, Richard's was worse. Red blood cell counts, blood sugar, cholesterol, electrolytes and digestive enzymes weren't optimum for either.

What YFH Recommended

The key to Tim's condition was zinc, magnesium and acidophilus. He added the proper bacteria and digestive enzymes, and he ate the right foods for his biology. In particular, his bowel couldn't tolerate raw vegetables, so he started eating only cooked vegetables. Although magnesium represented his greatest nutritional deficiency, he had to try a range of different magnesium formulations before he found one that his bowel could tolerate. Magnesium can make the stool looser.

Richard took most of the same supplements as Tim, but in greater quantities, especially magnesium. At our suggestion, he added additional fiber plus EPA fish oil, and eliminated the high carbohydrate foods that he'd previously been eating, which were completely wrong for his system.

Richard in particular had a weakened immune system, since his digestive tract was not able to extract the proper nutrients from food due to his poor digestion. As a dentist, patients were always breathing in his face, and he was constantly coming down with contagious illnesses. Additional zinc in his diet worked to balance his immune system and prevent this. Correcting the main digestive problem was also essential to strengthening his immune response.

Their Results

Within days of beginning customized YFH nutrition plans, both Richard and Tim found their digestive conditions improving rapidly, and eventually disappearing completely—for the first time ever! Tim's bloating, cramping and chronic diarrhea are no longer plaguing him, as long as he follows a proper diet and takes digestive enzymes as needed. Richard's constipation has also cleared up completely, and he finds that he can eat a broader range of foods than he ever would have dared try.

General Conclusions

This once again demonstrates that some people do well on one brand or formula of vitamin, and some do well on another. This is a function of individual biological variation. That's why Tim needed to try several magnesium formulations before finding one that was effective and that he could tolerate.

Some people are vitamin sponges—they need and can absorb large quantities—while others much more efficiently metabolize vitamins and, therefore, need smaller amounts. The only way to know what works for you is to re-test your blood to see the effect your current supplementation is having. If you're not achieving the proper result, you'll need to raise, lower or change your vitamin formulation, until your blood results demonstrate that you're hitting the optimum range. One additional complication: stress and illness tend to increase your body's need for nutrients. So if you go through a particularly trying time, or if you become sick, testing at this time can show you how your body is affected by stress. For instance, zinc levels can drop dramatically due to stress or illness. Once you see how low your zinc score drops under these conditions, you will have a better idea of how much to increase your zinc supplementation to compensate.

Tim Muldoon and Richard Krantz both had digestive disorders. When their systems were properly balanced, the men became more balanced. Muldoon's over-active bowel normalized. Dr. Krantz's under-active bowel normalized. Tim lost weight, Richard gained weight. Once again we see that when the body is properly nourished, various biological systems become balanced, and the body moves in the direction of optimum health.

Thyroid

Background
Jan Hurwitz (photo next page) is a physical education instructor who had always been in excellent health. When her mother developed kidney disease, she thought it prudent to do a complete set of preventive health tests.

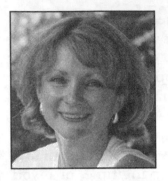

Her results came back negative for kidney disease.

The Problem

But, unfortunately, she discovered that she had thyroid disease. Her condition was serious, even though she hadn't yet begun to feel symptoms. Her doctor wanted to put her on Synthroid, a synthetic thyroid hormone which curtails the body's own production of thyroid hormones. Many people who begin taking Synthroid need to take it for the rest of their lives.

Jan was concerned about Synthroid's possible side effects. She told her doctor that she wanted to look for a natural solution before taking this drug. Her doctor said that his medical school training didn't include alternative health care, so he wouldn't know where she should even begin to look. But he encouraged her, and agreed to support a more natural approach. Her chiropractor told her he'd heard that YFH had a program for nourishing the thyroid to balance and restore its hormone output to optimum levels. So she called us.

Her YFH Blood Test Results

Our blood tests confirmed hypothyroidism—low thyroid hormone output and production. Her TSH score was 15.02, far above the laboratory normal reference range and her Free T4 test was abnormally low. Her zinc was low, her blood sugar was out of line (although not abnormal), her manual differential or detailed white blood cell tests were not optimum including her Bands test (a test for a specific type of white blood cell) which were elevated. (These tests are explained in Part III.)

What We Recommended

We told Jan that it takes time to improve thyroid function. She began by making changes in her diet. We recommended that she eat mainly low glycemic and low carbohydrate vegetables such as cauliflower and broccoli, with modest protein such as salmon or tofu. She also ate whole grain breads, nuts, yogurt and fruit in moderation. Her blood tests indicated a need to increase four different kinds of seaweed both in food and in supplements, as well as zinc, potassium, and B complex. And, of course, we continued to monitor her blood. As her levels of nutrients increased, she cut back on the supplements. She also worked to balance calcium. Our clinical work demonstrates that correcting thyroid problems helps to improve calcium absorption.

Her Results

By the end of her first year on the YFH program, her thyroid values had improved dramatically. Within eighteen months her thyroid values had returned to normal. When she told her doctor about the results, he was skeptical until he saw her test scores. But once he did, he was pleased and excited. He told her he'd never seen thyroid function return to normal solely as the result of proper nutrition. She continues to do well, and needless to say, does not need to take Synthroid.

General Conclusions

We applaud Jan's decision to do preventive testing, and to take active measures to correct her developing thyroid condition even before she detected physical symptoms. This made it much easier to fix the problem. However, continued testing is necessary to maintain optimum scores.

Whether a person has low or high thyroid function, the thyroid can rebalance and return to optimal hormonal output with proper nourishment provided the cells have not been irradiated, chemically killed, or surgically removed. Again, it's good to catch thyroid problems early. Is it possible to help people who have already been on Synthroid for years? Yes, but the healing process takes longer, and the prospect of complete success is reduced.

Thousands of people have developing thyroid disease and don't know it. They may not exhibit symptoms, and even if they do have their thyroid function tested, it's essential to do multiple tests over time to detect imbalances. Sometimes a test may fall within the normal range even when thyroid function is in decline. Without regular testing, it's not easy to know what is really going on.

A second problem in detecting thyroid disease early is that ranges considered normal for thyroid function have been continuously widened. Three years ago, the standard for a lab normal TSH (thyroid stimulating hormone) range was 0.4-4.0. Today it is 0.4-5.3. Some labs even consider 0.4-6.0 as normal as statistics are higher in their locale. So a year ago someone with a 4.8 TSH would have been flagged as having a thyroid problem. Today, that person would be considered within the lab normal range—for the sole reason that the lab normal range is broader than it used to be. Why is it broader? Because thyroid problems are ever more common across general populations, which means that labs are finding greater standard deviation of TSH results. And their bell curve lab normal ranges reflect that.

The bottom line? Everyone should do a set of five thyroid tests at least once a year. One of which should be the free T4, typically a very expensive test. Most doctors do not order this test because it is generally not covered by insurance.

Kids: Better Diets Are Better Than Drugs

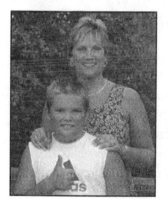

Background
Zach Alford was nine years old when YFH first met him. He lives in Maryland and is pictured with his mother Susan. As a toddler, he had shown signs of exceptional mental acuity.

The Problem
But as Zach grew into a young boy, he started developing processing-type problems. He was unable to focus on more than one thing at a time. He also had trouble with anything that required balance, like riding a bike. He started to lag behind the other kids in his classes. One of Zach's teachers told his parents she

suspected a learning disability, although she wasn't sure what it was. She recommended that he be tested.

Susan took Zach to a number of different specialists, including neurologists, psychiatrists and internists. The doctors came up with no common prognosis or treatment protocol. Susan was left without any answers. She was told that he may have Attention Deficit Disorder (ADD), that he simply needed to learn to live with his condition. She felt that putting him on psychotropic drugs would be too extreme. He stayed the same, but Susan was convinced that he could do better, and Zach desperately wanted to do better. So Susan committed herself to finding a solution. That's when she began working with YFH.

Zach's YFH Blood Tests

Most children have not yet developed the chronic medical problems reflected in the blood chemistries of the middle aged, but they can still be out of balance within a wide range of blood parameters. A supplement regimen was needed to balance Zach's various systems to compensate for his nutrient deficiencies. As a result, his blood sugar levels improved. He also eliminated most junk foods from his diet. He began eating more vegetables for snacks and more protein with fewer carbohydrates. However, children need more carbohydrates than adults.

His Results

Zach's condition improved, but not dramatically. From his blood tests, we knew that we'd suggested the right nutrition plan, so we began exploring other possibilities. We asked Susan if he'd ever suffered a fall. She had to think a while, but remembered that he'd fallen down the stairs once when he was younger. We suspected as much, and recommended that Susan take him to a chiropractor. For this problem, a special type of chiropractor called Atlas Orthogonal or upper cervical neck or Grostik method seem to work best. These new methods are precise, yet very gentle.

The chiropractor found a serious misalignment that YFH felt was both restricting Zach's neural responses and preventing nutrients from being properly utilized.

After his first adjustment, he began to improve rapidly. His mental acuity in classes was noticeably better, and he started getting A's. He had never been adept in sports, but now he was given an award for being one of the best players on the baseball team at school. He'd never been able to ride a bicycle, but now found it easy. He was able to think and write much more coherently. His parents felt that what made the difference for Zach was the chiropractic treatment, more than the customized nutrition plan YFH had developed for him.

But gradually his condition began to worsen. He responded less and less to his regular adjustments. His chiropractor began to investigate what had changed, and discovered that his family had become less strict in what they were allowing him to eat. Once he got back on the proper diet and supplements while continuing regular chiropractic adjustments, his condition began to improve, and he is again functioning well. In fact, his story was featured in *"Chicken Soup for the Chiropractic Soul"*.

General Conclusions

Proper nutrition can solve a much wider range of problems in children than is generally recognized. Most people know that too much sugar can cause normally well-behaved youngsters to become screaming banshees. But other deficiencies can also have dramatic effects on behavior.

For example, iron absorption rates significantly impact a child's ability to learn. Iron facilitates the transportation of oxygen to the cells of the body which are critical to mental acuity. The only way to know if your child is able to absorb iron in sufficient amounts is to do iron/ferritin tests. However, these tests are rarely ordered. It is assumed that children are healthy unless they exhibit extreme symptoms to the contrary. Most children are not tested unless they are sick, which makes their normal ranges actually sick ranges. This creates a broad lab normal reference range that is just not good enough.

Overall, comprehensive blood testing and evaluation give parents a blueprint to know which nutrients their child needs for optimum health.

Attention Deficit Disorder (ADD) diagnosis has recently become extremely common, especially in young children. But before taking such a serious step as putting your child on drugs, like Ritalin, why not be sure that there's not some simple solution related to their diet?

In the case of Zach, diet alone didn't solve his problem, but once we combined the right diet with the adjustment he needed after the fall he'd taken, his condition was corrected. The moral here? When one solution doesn't yield results, an open mind to other possible solutions may very well lead to success.

Immune System Disorders

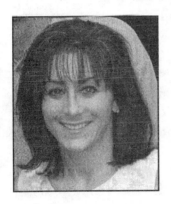

Background
Dr. Victoria Nassif is a dentist in Ohio.

Problem
When she was fourteen, Dr. Vicki Nassif contracted Toxic Shock Syndrome and was not expected to survive. She recovered, but her immune system was badly damaged and she was always sick. Later in her life she was forced to drop out of dental school for a year, due to debilitating migraines and was placed on antibiotics virtually full time to fight the colds, flu, and ear and throat infections that afflicted her constantly. She'd been examined by countless well-known migraine and immune system specialists, but none had been able to improve her condition. She told us that they all prescribed a range of drugs that did nothing but make her feel sicker. She heard about YFH and came to us to get her health back. In fact, she wanted to have another child, but having her first child was so debilitating that she knew she was not strong enough to try again.

Her YFH Blood Tests
It may surprise you to know that Vicki's blood test results fell entirely within the normal ranges used by most blood

labs and doctors. However, according to YFH's optimum ranges, her blood results didn't look normal at all. Vicki's thyroid, blood sugar, zinc, red blood cell count, hemoglobin, red blood cell morphology (size, shape and color of red blood cells) and manual differential (where the exact number of white blood cells are counted and reported by a professional) were all sub-optimum and out of balance.

What We Recommended

Vicki began rebuilding her immune system by increasing zinc, vitamin C, essential fatty acids, GLA (gamma linoleic acid), acidophilus, thyroid herbs and chromium chelate (balances pancreas and glucose tolerance factor). She also improved her tissue oxygenation and red blood cell count with B vitamins and more protein. She did blood testing every three months to make certain that she kept her blood chemistry profiles at precise optimum levels.

Her Results

Vicki's migraine headaches soon disappeared permanently. Her energy level improved, and she stopped catching every contagious illness making the rounds. Two years later, she was the healthiest she'd been since her early teenage years. Now she's better able to cope with the demands of a career and raising childen. Vicki's health improved so much that she was able to deliver a beautiful baby girl.

General Conclusions

Vicki's condition and resulting correction is proof positive that lab normal reference ranges are too wide to be used for early disease detection or to correct nutritional deficiencies. I must stress that without the three-month testing frequency, these results would not have been possible. When a suggestion is made to improve nutrition, the only way to know if it has worked is to retest. This is called fine-tuning. Without it, failure to correct the imbalance is inevitable.

Interpreting blood scores and working to bring them to much tighter optimum ranges through nutrition, Vicki was able to correct a debilitating illness that had plagued her for years.

Autoimmune Disorders/Arthritis

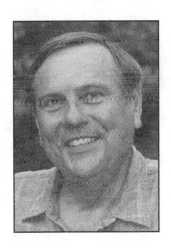

Background and Problem
Duke Shannahan is a senior executive who lives in Maryland. He'd occasionally had mild arthritis, an autoimmune disorder, but one day he got out of bed with tremendous pain in his joints. He decided he'd "tough" it out and loosen up his body by doing a few floor exercises. In excruciating pain, he went through his routine, and when he tried to get up, he couldn't move. He later found out that he'd had a major arthritic attack. Duke had been working with YFH for years, although recently he'd been extending the time between

his tests—so we hadn't been able to catch the downward slide in his blood chemistry that led to his attack.

His YFH Blood Tests

Duke's blood chemistry revealed all sorts of imbalances—just the sort of thing that can happen after an illness of some sort or major period of stress. His blood sugar level was much worse than usual, and his C-reactive protein was out of the optimum range along with his iron, red blood cells (RBCs), hemoglobin, calcium, magnesium and zinc. He confirmed that he'd been going through a particularly trying time with his company. He told us that he hadn't been too conscientious about his diet and reduced some supplements as well, since he had been feeling well. None of his scores, however, were out of the laboratory's normal reference range!

What We Recommended

Duke returned to his very strict eating program recommended by YFH for his condition. The high carbohydrates just had to go, as they are the major cause of irritation for Duke. He's Irish and potatoes are a problem—he hates to give them up, but they cause serious trouble for him every time he cheats. He increased his iron, zinc, calcium, magnesium and phosphorus—as well as vitamins E, A, C, B and essential fatty acids (EFA's)— the result of his blood test suggestions. In moments of high stress, Duke's zinc and iron especially need to be increased, as his body's demand for these minerals goes way up during arthritis attacks. A word of caution, please note: This must be proven with personal blood tests because everyone does not destroy iron and zinc due to stress. We recommended that Duke test every four months for a year or so to make sure that his scores didn't need to be readjusted.

Duke's Results

After a few months, Duke recovered completely, and turned over a new leaf as far as not taking his health for granted. He now tests his blood religiously at least three times a year. He doesn't follow the right diet quite so strictly, but he is much better than he was. He has regained full fluidity of movement and doesn't even suffer from minor arthritic pain or swelling. As long as he does not eat those potatoes and extra carbohydrates!

General Conclusions

Had Duke been receiving tests regularly before his attack, YFH would have undoubtedly detected the slide in his blood results, and could have recommended changes to diet and lifestyle that should have worked to prevent the attack. Arthritis sufferers can often achieve extremely good control of their condition with diet and stress management. The precision that blood testing offers in developing a diet optimized to one's own unique blood chemistry is generally more effective for control of arthritis than the general-purpose nutritional programs and the anti-inflammatory pill-popping regimen that many sufferers follow as well.

Rare Diseases

As discussed, to correct nutritional deficiencies that create symptoms, YFH's approach is to attempt to balance all known parameters of blood chemistry. Once we get the body's systems healthy, the body itself is often able to overcome even long-term and chronic illness and disease.

In over two decades of clinical work, YFH has seen that balancing the body's systems helps to strengthen the immune system. This can be effective for a vast range of medical conditions, even conditions for which medical knowledge is sparse. Both Lena's and Marcia's stories are examples of this.

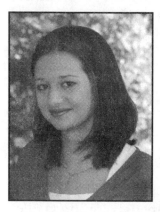

Background and Problem
Lena Wolfe was seventeen years old when we first tested her. Today she is in college pursuing a horticulture degree. She sidelines as a professional model with an agency in Cleveland. She has deep appreciation for being able to both work and study, because not long ago, it would have been impossible for her to do either. She has suffered for most of her life from a rare condition called Neurally Mediated Hypotension (NMH), as well as a reduced blood volume—about 28 percent less than normal. As a result, she had migraine headaches twenty-four hours a day, and would lose consciousness if she had to stand for more than about four minutes at a time. When we began working with her in 1999, she'd missed 135 days of school that year. She was being treated by a major research hospital and was heavily medicated on thirteen drugs. Her mother was terribly concerned, because the doctors

had said that if she missed taking her drugs for even one day, she'd go into cardiac arrest.

Her YFH Blood Tests

Lena is yet another sad example of the detriments of using broad ranges or "sick" blood ranges widely accepted as normal instead of more narrow optimum ranges. Why? Because all her blood tests fell within lab normal reference ranges, yet she was quite ill.

When evaluated according to the much narrower YFH optimum ranges, a number of problems became evident. She had a major blood sugar imbalance, severe protein and zinc deficiencies, thyroid problems, sodium and potassium imbalances, and a weak immune system.

What We Recommended

We gave Lena the tools she needed to balance her biological systems through diet and supplements—just as we do for all of our clients. When we customized her diet to her needs and biochemistry, the symptoms of her medical condition started becoming much less severe. Her headaches went away, she was able to go back to school, and she rarely has fainting spells.

General Conclusions

While we don't expect Lena's condition to ever be fully cured, optimizing her overall biological health provided dramatic improvements in her ability to lead a normal life. She knows that her active lifestyle causes many changes in her blood chemistry and nutritional needs, so she has vowed to test frequently for the rest of her life.

Learn more about Lena by visiting our Website at www.yourfuturehealth.com.

Marcia's Story

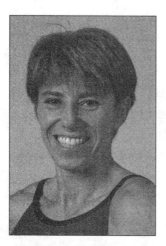

Background

Marcia is the founder of a highly respected physical fitness program called *Boot Camp Bodies.* She competed in the X-Games for Inline Downhill Speed Skating, and the World Games for Speed Skating. She was inducted into the Roller Skating Hall of Fame, won many national titles, and broke four previously held records during the Inline-Skating Nationals of 1974. To commemorate her victories Marcia's skating coach gave her a plaque inscribed, "May God give you the strength in life as He did in the races."

When Marcia was only 25, her mother died. But she can still hear her mother's words of wisdom: "If you don't have your health, you have nothing." This message and the words of her coach were to take on deep, personal significance. In 2003, she developed a serious circulatory problem that suddenly made walking nearly impossible. She was told the horrifying news that her toes might have to be amputated. This would be devastating for anyone. In her case, her livelihood depended on optimum health – on being at the top of her game.

What frustrated Marcia was that she was confident she ate well. She knew she exercised sufficiently (and then some). She said, "How could this possibly happen?"

The Problem

Marcia's symptoms included blood clots and ulcer-like lesions on her toes. Her feet were yellow on the bottom and at times also red, swollen, purple, numb, and cold. Her hair was limp and lifeless, her fingernails stopped growing, and her skin was rough; nicks and small paper cuts would not heal. Her hands were so swollen every morning that she could barely flex her fingers. Her joints ached. Her legs and arms ached. She could barely get out of bed much less contemplate teaching her Boot Camp Bodies classes. She said that she felt a hundred years old. But unlike Methuselah she felt she was dying inside.

She spent five days in a hospital, where she had every test imaginable. She was checked for leukemia, Parkinson's, diabetes, arthritis, multiple sclerosis, lupus, plus every other autoimmune disease possible. Although her doctors were compassionate, they were unable to identify the cause for her mysterious illness. They said she "defied diagnosis."

Finally, she was told that she had protein S deficiency which is irreversible. She was instructed to take coumadin (a blood thinner) to help dissolve the clots, and was sent home.

Fortunately, Marcia remembered meeting my son Brian, who told her about YFH several months earlier. When modern medicine had nothing to offer by way of a solution, she turned to nutrition for help.

Her YFH Blood Tests

Marcia needed a Basic HealthPrint plus the following additional tests: the heart package including a VAP genetic cholesterol density measurement, C-Reactive Protein, Homocysteine, and Omega 3 Profile+, Ferritin, Progesterone, Thyroid Panel, and the female cancer package including CA-125, CA-15-3, CEA, and CA19-9. Although her scores were within the normal range, a myriad of nutritional deficiencies were evident in her blood. Immediate changes to her diet and supplement plan were needed.

What We Recommended

Marcia's glucose or blood sugar level was too high for her. When the test scores were comprehensively reviewed and compared, rather than looked at individually, early stage diabetes was apparent. She was producing insulin erratically. She did not oxygenate her tissue well. Marcia's iron, hemoglobin, red blood cells and ferritin tests were not optimum for her. These imbalances prevented her from getting oxygen inside the cells. In fact, her cells were dying from lack of oxygen. Again, let us remember that all of these scores were considered normal.

Her circulatory and immune systems were far from being up to par. Her blood was moving very slowly due to an overload of platelets across areas of plaque buildup on the inside of her blood vessels. This plaque build up developed because she had super-dense cholesterol, practically no EPA fish oil and excess glucose. Traditional testing, however, showed none of this. (In fact, all of her cholesterol, triglyceride and glucose scores by traditional testing were interpreted as fantastic.)

The Omega 3 Profile+ test (that looks for inflammation, immune strength and risk of cardiovascular disease) showed severe essential fatty acid deficiencies and an excess of arachidonic acid. Her Omega 3 Score (a measure of cardiac risk) was 2.8. An adequate score is 7.2. For Marcia, however, a safer score would be closer to 15. Her AA/EPA ratio (measures silent inflammation) was 20.59— one of the worst scores I had ever seen. For perspective a good serum AA/EPA ratio is 1.5. However, Marcia's genetics and other test responses, indicated that a lower AA/EPA score would be more appropriate. The specific AA/EPA target score could only be determined by retesting.

No wonder she was in so much pain! Oxygen could not get to the cells, waste could not be removed, her platelets made her blood thick and her glucose level was high enough to make her blood sweet and sticky. The combination of imbalances caused the clots. She needed a total diet overhaul.

The saddest part of Marcia's story is her problems did not develop overnight—they had been developing since birth. Had she tested preventively, before she experienced symptoms, her problems very likely could have been managed or even avoided—saving her severe pain, suffering and expense. The advantage of tracking test scores consistently is that you can usually see disease brewing in time to correct the imbalances *before* symptoms occur.

Her Results

YFH does not diagnose, treat or cure disease, nor does it sell supplements. The specific nutrients that Marcia required were identified from her YFH blood tests. Our specialty is to pinpoint the problem nutritionally and provide data that allows you to discuss your health issues with your health professional. This is the best possible way to take the necessary tried-and-true health-embracing actions.

In Marcia's case, she began eating a low carbohydrate and low glycemic (or low insulin-producing) diet. This gave her pancreas a chance to "rest," and reduced her high arachidonic acid level. She added high-quality food supplements, including B-complex, vitamin E, chelated chromium (with glucose tolerance factor), Coenzyme Q-10, acidophilus, vitamin C, zinc, lysine, GLA, lecithin, calcium and magnesium. As a result of her omega 3 essential fatty acid deficiency, she also supplemented her diet with massive quantities of EPA fish oil.

Her diet was changed to include more nutrient-dense food intake. She only used supplements where there was an extreme deficiency. Her doctor agreed that she did not need the coumadin medication. Marcia was relieved to be able to discontinue the medication. She continued to be clot free using only the diet and supplements.

Within one month, Marcia's color came back and her hair was beautiful again. The best result, however, was that her pain subsided completely, her joints returned to normal, and the ulcers on her toes that threatened amputation were gone. Within three months she regained all her strength and happily reports that her workouts are better than ever.

We believe symptom improvements are important, but test evidence is even better. Marcia was retested six months after she began her new dietary program to confirm that she was on the right track. Now her Omega 3 Score registered 15.74, up from a dangerous 2.81. Her AA/EPA went down from 20.59 to 1.10. In all, over 35 scores were optimized including glucose, iron, red blood cells, hemoglobin, ferritin, uric acid, globulin, bands, and LDL cholesterol. This led to better oxygenation, waste removal, cardiovascular health and immune systems strength.

The new analysis confirmed that other than the iron, which rose a bit too high, Marcia made the right changes to her nutritional program. Her doctors were thrilled to see her progress. Although people may experience improvement, the tests may confirm that they have not quite achieved the right balance, as with her iron retest. Retesting can affirm the progress, or lack of it.

Marcia was interviewed on CBS and Fox news just six months after the onset of her illness. She was filmed doing one of her workouts, including running the steps at the University of Cincinnati football stadium. I am grateful to Marcia for her insistence to share her incredible testimonial publicly and for the credit she gave my company and to me. She says that the YFH system saved her life. Personally, I think that she saved her own life. YFH pointed her in the right direction, but she had the determination to make the changes. She has become a prominent spokesperson for preventive blood testing, and now validates her lifestyle changes regularly with the YFH highly scientific measurements and evaluations.

General Conclusions

For Marcia, as with most of us, results that appeared normal with standard analyses, simply weren't good enough. They were far from optimum! The disease that came without warning due to nutritional deficiencies disappeared completely within three months once Marcia knew exactly what she needed to do to rebalance her system. She is a perfect example of why I titled this book, *"Normal Blood Test Scores Aren't Good Enough!"*

Multiple Diseases & Treatment Complications

Background and Problem

Ginni Shaner (photo next page) contracted Hepatitis C (a liver disease that has no known cure) from a blood transfusion. She was treated with chemotherapy, which resulted in damage to her immune system. In particular, her red blood cell count dropped dramatically and her

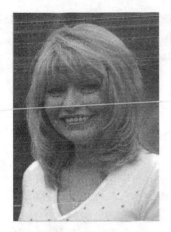

body lost its ability to make blood platelets. She was retaining fluids and was tremendously bloated. She was also diabetic. The prognosis from her doctors was extremely poor. They told her that there was nothing more they could do, and that she should begin getting her affairs in order. Then Ginni came to YFH.

Ginni's YFH Blood Tests and Our Recommendations

Ginni had been on a diet that was only adding to her problems. She'd been told to avoid protein and was eating nothing but carbohydrates and buttermilk. YFH suggested a high protein diet, with only low glycemic and low carbohydrate vegetables, 1-2 slices of bread, olive oil plus 1 piece of fresh fruit daily eaten in the evening only. Among other benefits, this helped control her blood sugar. Ginni decided to take extra amounts of vitamins C, E and B, zinc, magnesium, calcium, and essential fatty acids to balance her blood test levels. She nourished her thyroid with seaweed supplements.

General Conclusions

Given the poor prognosis from her doctors, we're very pleased to report that Ginni improved rapidly. The fluid retention disappeared and she lost four dress sizes. Ginni is no longer diabetic. Her liver is showing signs of healing itself, with scores improved by fifty percent. Her body is again making platelets! She's now able to hold down a full-time job, and recently graduated from college. She has tons of energy and her doctors consider her recovery nearly miraculous. Ginni herself considers it a miracle, and attributes it both to the YFH program and the healing power of prayer.

Boost Energy and Overcome Fatigue

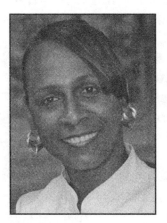

Eloise Allen is a schoolteacher, so she needs to be able to keep up with her students. But she increasingly got headaches and found herself exhausted. Her regular physicals never indicated health problems. Nevertheless, her fatigue continued. She needed a major diet adjustment and her problems were the lack of zinc, overproduction of insulin and abnormal size and color of her red blood cells. She could not properly supply oxygen to her cells.

Her HealthPrint indicated that she needed additional B vitamins, iron, chromium with GTF and protein. She also needed zinc, but was unable to tolerate zinc supplements, so she added large amounts of organic cinnamon to her diet, which raised her zinc level almost immediately. She recovered from her exhaustion and headaches, and is now feeling great.

Keeping Cancer at Bay

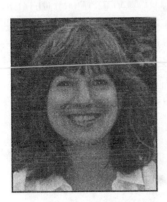

Joyce Weston has an active outdoor life focused on horse training. She has an extensive history of cancer in her family on her father's side, and diabetes on her mother's side. Her father died of cancer and her sister has been battling cancer for several years. To reduce her risk factors, she uses her HealthPrint to optimize her diet and supplement choices, and to keep track of the beginning of any decline in her blood chemistry, so that she is able to treat any developing medical condition early. Joyce has been testing her blood for years. Her results are usually excellent—she follows a proper diet religiously, but every now and then we find something that requires correction.

Avoiding Side Effects of Harsh Drugs

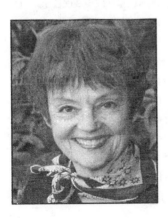

Dr. Jane Dodson has an even greater genetic propensity for cancer—her sisters are all on strong cancer-prevention drugs. She does a full HealthPrint, CEA, CA-125 and CA-15-3 predictive cancer tests every four months. (These tests are described in Part III of this book.) She's tested with YFH for more than nineteen years, and by continually

129

optimizing her nutrition from HealthPrint data, she has avoided both anti-cancer drugs and any symptoms of the disease. She reports that she hasn't had so much as a cold in more than a decade. She carefully monitors her zinc levels and uses supplements to keep zinc blood serum in the optimum range. In her sixties, she runs a busy dental practice and is full of life. She's an excellent example for us all.

Winning at Prostate Management

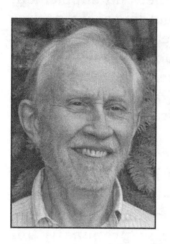 Hal Kerber is eighty years old, in excellent health, and began working with YFH as a way to sort out all the confusing health advice he was hearing. He felt that basing his lifestyle choices on an analysis of his own blood chemistry would be the most reliable way to guarantee that he was doing the right things for his biochemistry, regardless of what worked for others. Since most older men are at risk for prostate trouble, he was particularly interested in what YFH could discover in this area. He tested both total PSA (prostate cancer test) and Free Percent PSA (Free Percent PSA range is 1-100 percent. Higher is better.) His first total PSA score was 2.8—within the lab normal reference range, but not considered optimum. We recommended that he increase his protein intake. He supplemented his diet with B vitamins, saw palmetto and zinc. His second total PSA

test a year later was an outstanding 1.35. Hal is proof positive that, contrary to what many men are told, PSA scores do not necessarily need to keep going up with age. The right diet and supplement program can lower PSA scores and keep them down.

Really Winning at Prostate Management

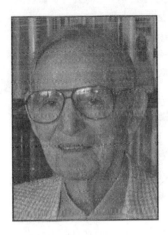

Harold Miller will be ninety years old this fall. He's a Hilton Hotel landlord, and MIT graduate. He's achieved extraordinary success over a long and diverse career, but he had a rude shock.

During one of his regular YFH HealthPrints, Harold's total PSA score, which had always been optimum, suddenly registered a worrisome 12.8. His corresponding Free Percent PSA score was only 18 percent. Because he tests regularly, he knew that these scores were not even in the laboratory normal reference range.

Harold is a long-term client of YFH. We felt these results were serious, so we strongly recommended he see a specialist immediately. He was told that elevated PSA scores were a normal part of getting old. We suggested that he get a second opinion and he decided to make an appointment with Dr. Robert Atkins at the celebrated

Center of Complementary Medicine, founded by Dr. Atkins, in New York City.

Dr. Atkins recommended two specific supplements, which (along with YFH dietary recommendations) brought Harold's PSA scores back to optimum range. Within three months his total PSA had dropped to 7.51, and his Free Percent PSA rose to 20. After another three months his total PSA had dropped to an exceptional level of 1, while Free Percent rose to 39. Harold improved because of his diet and supplements. He used neither prostate drugs nor radiation treatments.

Recovering and Thriving

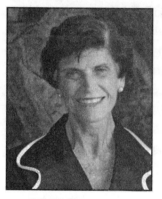

Ruth Bird is eighty-six years old. Over twenty years ago, Ruth was afflicted with colon cancer and later developed cervical cancer. Initially she was treated for cancer, and a portion of her colon was removed, but her prognosis was not good. Ruth's family was told that she had only six months to live because sixteen of seventeen biopsies were positive for cancer.

But no one had told Ruth! Her family had little faith in nutrition and positive thinking. But Ruth defied them all. She recovered from her cancers and then later began working with YFH to develop a customized nutrition plan to detect any reappearance of cancer and to improve oxygenation of her cells and her cholesterol scores. Ruth says, "No sense dying of cardiovascular disease when you have beaten cancer." To the surprise of her family and doctors, the cancer did not reappear, and it has been more than *twenty years* since then. Today, Ruth plays tennis twice a week, remains quite active, and does her YFH HealthPrint at very regular intervals.

General Conclusions

Have you detected a pattern yet concerning what our clients have done to correct a wide range of physical symptoms? Working to balance all of our biological systems is the key.

What varies from person to person are in the recommended specific foods, formulations and amounts of supplements, and fine-tuning of the person's customized plan done by retesting. This customization is what I feel makes a YFH HealthPrint more effective than even the best general-purpose dietary and wellness programs.

Preventive Health

I've occasionally explained to someone I've just met what YFH does, and the usual response is that they know someone who's ill whom they believe would love to do a YFH HealthPrint.

My answer is always the same. I point out that although our program benefits those who are ill, the benefit is even greater for those who are healthy. We've helped hundreds of people correct scores due to serious afflictions, but the YFH program is even more effective for keeping the healthy, well, healthy. So if this describes you, I encourage you not only to give this book to an ill friend or family member, but to consider taking into account what preventive blood testing can do for you.

I mentioned earlier that one of the best things preventive blood testing offers is tracking of slides in your health before a serious debilitating disease surfaces. We know of no better way to identify and correct developing illness in the earliest, most treatable stage. Human biochemistry is diverse, and everyone responds to lifestyle choices and stresses in different ways. So there's no telling if you're someone who has enough health to be able to live into old age, or if your biology is such that you'll need to begin improving your diet and lifestyle by the time you reach your thirties.

Let me emphasize that point again. Some people can get away with unhealthy diets and lifestyle longer than others due to their biochemical predisposition. The body can take it for only so long, and then the decline comes rapidly.

It's essential to track these declines by tracking your changes in blood chemistry. That's the best way to know when you can no longer get away with burning the candle at both ends. This is the point at which you need to get serious about making lifestyle choices for the better. If not, this may be the point at which you'll start losing your health.

The Final Word

It's hard not to be convinced about how powerful preventive blood testing can be for increasing the quality and span of your life—especially when the tests are repeated regularly, and interpreted properly.

I encourage you and those you love to begin having regular preventive blood testing. The cost is low and the benefits priceless.

Whatever your path, we at YFH wish you a life of vigorous health and an ongoing sense of fulfilled well-being.

Essential Blood Test
Reference Guide

Blood Test Table of Contents

Hundreds of different blood tests are available. The tests listed below are essential for general illness prevention and early identification of the onset of disease. They are also useful for addressing specific problems such as male and female cancers.

Electrolytes

Minerals

Bones

Kidneys

Thyroid

Special Tests

The following pages explain these tests and their significance for optimum health.

1. Sodium

Without sodium, your body could not carry nutrients and wastes to and from cells, transmit electrical impulses throughout your nervous system, give you control of your voluntary bodily movements, or support the automatic functions of your intestinal tract.

Sodium helps balance water volume and pressure in body tissues. Because sodium acts as a sponge, it prevents water from overloading cells by keeping the water in the bloodstream and in the fluids that surround cells.

People with high blood pressure are often put on low-sodium diets because increased sodium also causes increased water volume, which raises pressure on the cell walls and can cause high blood pressure. Too much sodium can also result in edema, an increase in the fluid surrounding the cells. Edema is indicated by swollen ankles and/or swelling (bloating) in other parts of the body.

A sodium test helps to determine if you have any salt or electrolyte imbalances in your body. An imbalance could be related to possible kidney and/or adrenal-gland disorders.

A score above the Lab Reference Range may suggest:
- Water retention and weight gain
- High blood pressure
- Adrenal gland dysfunction
- Dehydration (which may be caused by not drinking enough water)
- Diabetes

A score below the Lab Reference Range may suggest:
- Damage to the adrenal glands/Addison's disease
- Cirrhosis of the liver
- Damage to kidneys/severe diabetes
- Congestive heart failure / use of diuretic drugs

- Hypothyroidism
- Excessive diarrhea or sweating

2. Potassium

Potassium is the major mineral component inside body cells. It is essential for muscle contraction, and since your heart is a muscle, it would not beat without potassium. Nerve fibers also rely on potassium as a conductor for electric impulses.

Order a potassium test if you experience:
- Muscular weakness, cramps, and general lethargy, which could be symptoms of insufficient potassium. If a low potassium level continues over an extended period, the result could be partial paralysis of the hands and legs and interference with your heartbeat
- High blood pressure, especially if you are receiving diuretic medications
- Weight gain and bloating

A score above the Lab Reference Range may suggest:
- Pounding of the heart, especially when in a prone position
- Heart attack danger, if the level is very high over a prolonged time
- The possibility of a false score, which occurs when a sample is not handled properly
- Adrenal exhaustion

A score below the Lab Reference Range may suggest:
- Heart beat irregularities

143

- Loss of body fluids
- Weight gain due to retained fluids
- Stress
- Exhaustion
- Depletion from diuretic drugs
- Swollen ankles, fingers
- Exaggerated PMS and menopause symptoms
- Partial paralysis of hands and legs
- Side effect of blood pressure drug depletion

3. Chloride

Chloride helps the body remain in a state of electrical neutrality. Chloride is also the companion component to sodium, which forms sodium chloride or salt.

Consider running a chloride test if:
- You have experienced excessive sweating, diarrhea, or vomiting for several days
- You have just had surgery, especially intestinal surgery, or have experienced situations in which intravenous fluids are the major source of nutrients and minerals

A score above the Lab Reference Range may indicate:
- Water loss without adequate replacement, which is common in those with diabetes
- Excessive use of ammonium chloride expectorants
- Hyperventilation
- Increased chlorine in your water source
- A need to clean your drinking water filter

A score below the Lab Reference Range may indicate:
- The adrenal gland deficiency known as Addison's disease
- Intestinal obstruction
- Metabolic acidosis common in those with diabetes

4. Carbon Dioxide as Bicarbonate

You probably learned in high school biology that the oxygen you use in your body is changed into carbon dioxide in your lungs and exchanged for a new supply of oxygen. But before that can happen, red blood cells convert the carbon dioxide into bicarbonate, the same chemical compound as the baking soda in your kitchen cupboard.

Carbon dioxide can be out of balance because of hypoventilation (breathing too slowly) or hyperventilation (breathing too rapidly). Hypoventilation, or inadequate exchange of air, can be caused by fluid in your lungs or by drugs that affect the breathing control center of your brain. Increased bicarbonate in blood is called respiratory acidosis and can produce coma and death. Hyperventilation is caused by losing too much carbon dioxide through rapid breathing. This low level of carbon dioxide is called respiratory alkalosis and is marked by hand and foot spasms and a sense of being suffocated.

A score above the Lab Reference Range may suggest:
- Hypoventilation or inadequate exchange of air
- Low oxygen

- Increased ingestion of alkaline foods or licorice
- Inadequate exercise

A score below the Lab Reference Range may suggest:
- Hyperventilation (breathing too rapidly)
- Hysteria/Anxiety
- Fever
- Increased ketones or acetones from fasting or diabetes
- Diarrhea
- Kidney disease
- Central nervous system disease

5. Glucose

Glucose is the basic fuel for all your bodily functions, both physical and intellectual. We know glucose by its more familiar name, sugar. Pure sugars, like sucrose and fructose (or simple carbohydrates), are absorbed quickly by your body; complex carbohydrates, like beans, bread or rice, are absorbed more slowly and must be broken down before they can be absorbed.

Insulin rapidly removes sugar from your blood and moves it into your cells. Insulin is a hormone secreted by the pancreas. It stimulates the formation of glycogen, a form of glucose that is suitable for storage in the body, primarily in the liver. The body uses the reserved glycogen at times when your muscles need more energy than is available from blood glucose. For example, reserved glycogen is used when you do not eat for long periods of time or if you do extreme exercise, like running a marathon. Excess glucose that is not needed for your reserves ends up stored as fat. When you consistently eat more calories than you need, the calories cannot be utilized and are not needed for reserves, therefore the glucose is stored as fat. Eating small meals is a better technique when you want to lose weight. (You burn more calories that way.) But, as we all know, this is not easy to achieve.

Diabetes is caused by inadequate insulin secretion or inefficient insulin metabolism. Since insulin removes sugar from your blood, an inadequate supply means a high blood sugar level remains in your body tissues.

Possible causes of secondary diabetes (hyperglycemia) with an under-production of insulin are:
- Acromegaly, an excess of growth hormone
- Overactive thyroid, or adrenal glands
- Liver malfunction

The opposite case is hypoglycemia (low blood sugar) with an over-production of insulin. Possible causes of hypoglycemia may be:
- Inadequate cortisol secretion (a hormone controlled by the adrenal gland) and stress
- Improper functioning of the liver or pancreas

A score above the Lab Reference Range indicates:
- Diabetes or high blood sugar with an under-production of insulin. (See your doctor!) The pancreas needs a rest from eating too many sugars that require insulin. If you rest your pancreas by reducing the need for insulin, the insulin balance can be restored.

See Dr. Kramer's case study.

A score below the Lab Reference Range indicates:
- Hypoglycemia or low blood sugar with an over-production of insulin from too many sugars or carbohydrates in the diet.

6. Phosphorus

Phosphorus works with calcium to form an insoluble combination that gives your skeleton its shape and strength. In return, your skeleton serves as a major reservoir of phosphorus, which neutralizes excess acid in the blood. The 10 - 20 percent of phosphorus not stored in the bones is found in the soft tissues where it is required for carbohydrate metabolism and muscle contraction.

Found in most food, phosphorus is easily absorbed from the gastrointestinal tract and quickly put to use in the body. After a meal, the phosphorus gets busy helping transport sugar molecules from the bloodstream to the body's cells. The average diet usually provides enough phosphorus or too much, but rarely too little.

A score above the Lab Reference Range may indicate:
- Kidney disease
- Kidney stones, an insoluble form of calcium and phosphorous deposits in tissues formed when levels of both are too high

A score below the Lab Reference Range may indicate:
- Inadequate absorption of phosphorus, perhaps

through frequent use of antacids like Tums
- Inadequate dietary intake of phosphorus
- Diarrhea
- Poor bone formation

7. Calcium

Calcium is the most plentiful mineral in your body and plays a highly diversified role. Your bones and teeth are made up of and store approximately 99 percent of your calcium. The remaining one percent is called "free calcium" and is dissolved in your bloodstream. Despite the small quantity, this dissolved calcium is of critical importance because it:
- Maintains bone strength
- Facilitates muscle contraction
- Aids nerve impulse transmission
- Helps blood to clot

To understand how calcium works, think of your bones as a coral reef and your body fluids as the sea, continually building and changing in structure. When the level of free calcium falls below the minimum normal level, your body sets off a series of alarm reactions to remedy the situation. This results in a hormone produced by the parathyroid gland (PTH) which:
- Frees calcium from the bones
- Enhances the return of calcium from the kidneys
- Stimulates production of active vitamin D

It is necessary to have enough calcium but be careful not to take too much. If you have a very high level of calcium from supplementation and not enough magnesium and B complex for balance, you may develop kidney stones. If you need more of each, take your magnesium and B in the morning and your calcium in the evening and watch your alkaline phosphatase score go down as the magnesium helps calcium utilization. The two can fight for entry into the cells when taken together in equal amounts.

A score above the Lab Reference Range may indicate:
- Hyperactive functioning of the parathyroid gland
- Too much vitamin D

A score below the Lab Reference Range may indicate:
- Parathyroid and thyroid gland deficiencies
- Kidney disorder
- Intestines have difficulty absorbing nutrients
- Vitamin D deficiency

8. Magnesium

Magnesium is another major mineral with a large essential role for balanced body functions. The exact amount of magnesium required has not been determined, and some people get sufficient magnesium through diet, especially from vegetables and meat. Peanuts and shrimp are excellent sources of magnesium. When tested, most people find their levels too low in relation to their calcium levels. Testing reveals that magnesium levels may be too low when compared with their high intake of calcium. Raising magnesium intake should lower the calcium level in your blood by forcing the calcium inside the bones and muscle tissue, a desired result.

Maintaining a proper balance between calcium and magnesium is very important. Magnesium activates your parathyroid hormone needed to regulate calcium levels in your blood. People on diuretic therapy requiring potassium should also be alert for magnesium deficiency. (Potassium therapy without magnesium replacement is usually ineffective.) YFH finds low magnesium levels in 90 percent of clients tested. I'm convinced that magnesium tests are critical to help prevent osteoporosis, an irregular heart beat, or fibromyalgia, even though this test is not a part of any standard panel of tests suggested by the American Medical Association.

A score above the Lab Reference Range may indicate:
- Magnesium toxicity, which acts as a sedative and can cause the heart to stop beating
- Kidney malfunction
- Dehydration
- Adrenal deficiency

A score below the Lab Reference Range may indicate:
- Improper diet
- Treatment with intravenous fluids
- Excessive diarrhea or vomiting
- Neuromuscular difficulties such as twitching or quivering
- Irritability caused by noise or visual stimulation
- Ineffective utilization of calcium

9. Zinc

Zinc is a mineral with a key role in maintaining a healthy body. It activates enzymes that metabolize proteins, nucleic acids and other vital bodily processes.
Zinc is involved in the production and storage of insulin in the pancreas. In addition, it helps maintain healthy skin tissue and is, therefore, part of the therapy used for patients suffering from extensive burns.

Although zinc is not considered an aphrodisiac, it is involved in the production of testosterone. It is also essential for the proper functioning of the prostate gland and sperm production. YFH has found a low level of zinc in most of our clients who suffer from low libido and infertility. In general, 80 percent of our clients are low in zinc. Like so many other nutrients, too much zinc can be just as harmful as too little.

You should test for zinc to check your:
- Immune system
- Prostate/Reproductive organs
- Wound healing, eye health, skin disorders
- Pancreas (blood sugar)

A score above the Lab Reference Range may indicate:
- Over-stimulation of the immune system
- A need to retest (unless excessive supplementation is the cause)

A score below the Lab Reference Range may indicate or result in:

- Diabetes in adults
- Delayed healing of skin/acne/psoriasis
- Reduced ability to taste or smell food
- Retarded growth in children of both sexes
- Improper functioning of the prostate gland
- Infertility
- Weak immune system
- A need for dietary increase of zinc
- Advancing macular degeneration
- Failure of male pubertal development

10. Iron

Iron is present in minuscule amounts in your blood, but without it you couldn't live. Seventy percent of the iron in your body is contained in the oxygen-carrying part of the red blood cells called hemoglobin. Iron is a recycling wonder. Your body absorbs only 10 percent of the iron you consume. Much of the rest is recycled and re-synthesized through a protein called transferrin. When red blood cells break down, transferrin takes iron from the hemoglobin, stores it in various places in the body and then transports it to the bone marrow to help in the process of manufacturing new red blood cells.

Consider testing for your iron level if you:
- Use oral contraceptives
- Have excessive menstrual bleeding
- Have cancer, kidney disease, or rheumatoid arthritis
- Have chronic blood loss
- Have insufficent intake of iron-rich foods
- Are chronically tired

A score above the Lab Reference Range may indicate:
- Use of oral contraceptives or lead poisoning
- Accelerated breakdown of red blood cells
- Decreased formation of fresh red blood cells
- A defect in your iron's ability to combine with hemoglobin
- Consumption of too much well water (or a dirty water filter)

A score below the Lab Reference Range may indicate:
- Chronic blood loss in the intestinal tract, possibly due to hiatal hernia, an ulcer, or intestinal parasites
- Decreased iron absorption
- Excessive menstrual bleeding
- Infection
- Chronic kidney disease
- Cancer
- Stress (physical, mental, or environmental)
- Pregnancy
- Vitamin C deficiency
- Rheumatoid arthritis

11. Alkaline Phosphatase

Highly concentrated in your bones and liver and to a lesser extent in your spleen, kidneys and intestines, alkaline phosphatase enzymes can be an important indicator of liver or bone damage. An elevated level of this enzyme in the bloodstream alerts doctors to possible disorders of these major organ systems. If this score is elevated above the Lab Reference Range, be sure to review the results with your doctor.

Elevated levels of alkaline phosphatase could also indicate increased bone cell activity in children whose bones are still growing (sudden increase may indicate a growth spurt) and in people whose bones are mending from fractures. Growth spurts and trauma may cause alkaline phosphatase enzymes to be released into the blood in large amounts.

The degree of elevation of alkaline phosphatase enzymes, combined with other blood chemistry, can help in the diagnosis of major organ diseases. An elevation that emerges suddenly, even if the score remains within the lab normal reference range, should be investigated unless the patient is a growing child or is someone who has recently undergone a fracture.

A score above the Lab Reference Range may indicate:
- Bone diseases such as rickets
- Metastatic cancers from other tissues
- Parathyroid gland activity
- Liver disease
- Gallbladder disease
- Pancreatic cancer
- Osteoporosis

A score below the Lab Reference Range may indicate:
- Anorexia or severe malnutrition if the range is less than 15

It is not unusual for a score less than the Lab Reference Range to be normal/healthy for many people. This is because the people in the control group, upon whom the

Laboratory Reference Range is based, often do not have optimum health (and typically will have higher scores).

12. Blood Urea Nitrogen (BUN)

BUN is the result of protein breakdown in your body. Proteins are reduced to amino acids, which are converted to carbon dioxide, water and ammonia. Since ammonia is a poison, your liver converts it to urea, which is then dissolved in your blood, carried to your kidneys and eliminated. However, because urea is a small molecule, it is capable of cell membrane penetration and appears in saliva, perspiration, intestinal fluids and brain and spinal cord fluids. An increase of protein in the diet can produce an ammonia-like body odor smell. It is critical to increase water intake if you are on a high protein diet to help flush protein waste from your kidneys.

BUN levels in your body are primarily affected by:
- The amount of protein in your diet
- The rate of protein breakdown in your body
- Your kidneys' ability to excrete urea

A score above the Lab Reference Range may suggest:
- A high protein diet
- Dehydration or lack of water intake
- Kidney problems
- Congestive heart failure
- Edema (swelling due to imbalance of electrolytes)
- Internal hemorrhage
- Infections
- Cancer

- Drug utilization
- Increased thyroid activity
- Uncontrolled diabetes
- Urinary tract problems

A score below the Lab Reference Range may suggest:
- Severe protein malnutrition
- Excessive water intake
- Cirrhosis of the liver

Below normal BUN readings are rare.

13. Creatinine

Creatinine results from the breakdown of creatinine phosphate, which works with other body substances to form energy to make your muscles work. The waste material created by this process is called creatinine.

Creatinine is extemely useful as an indicator of how well your kidneys are functioning. The level should remain relatively constant and is perhaps your best indicator of kidney health. Elevation beyond your Personal Normal level may suggest overworked kidneys. This score is not affected by the amount of protein you eat as is the case with your Blood Urea Nitrogen (BUN) score. Nor does your water intake affect this score. However, a common body-building supplement known as creatine (not creatinine) may have its impact on this score. More testing is needed to confirm whether the positive physical enhancement is actually healthy for one's body.

When your creatinine level is in the normal range, your kidneys are doing their job of filtering and excreting toxic wastes. This score will generally not rise above the Lab Reference Range until both kidneys are not working properly. An increasing score can help detect kidney problems early, and can be a harbinger of potential kidney problems.

A score above the Lab Reference Range may indicate:
- Damage to kidneys' ability to filter and remove waste from the bloodstream
- Reduced blood flow to kidneys caused by poor circulation or blood clots
- Malfunction of both kidneys

A score below the Lab Reference Range may indicate:
- Low energy level
- Inability to make the muscles work properly

14. BUN/Creatinine Ratio

The BUN/creatinine ratio is used to determine how well your kidneys are functioning. The creatinine level is relatively stable, so it is the Blood Urea Nitrogen score that makes the ratio fluctuate. This ratio is dependent on how much protein you consume and the quantity of water you drink. If you have too little water or too much protein, your score will be higher. To determine the ratio, divide the BUN level by the creatinine level.

A score above the Lab Reference Range may indicate:
- A kidney or kidneys that are overloaded with waste

- Kidney failure that can occur with diabetes
- Medication or drug overload/reaction

A score below the Lab Reference Range may indicate:
- An imbalance of the BUN level to the creatinine level
- Inability to make the muscles work properly

15. Uric Acid

Gout, a disease that has been joked about for centuries, is the result of elevated uric acid in the body. When this disease is present, uric acid is deposited near cartilage tissues. Microcrystals form in the fluids within the joints to cause such an attack. The condition is very painful and includes swelling of the joint. Sometimes a crystal actually bursts through the skin during an attack, usually affecting the big toe.

Gout is a metabolic disorder resulting from either the increased production of uric acid in the body or the decreased elimination of uric acid through the kidneys.

Uric acid results from the breakdown of nucleic acids (formed of carbohydrates, phosphoric acid and nitrogen), which are complex molecules that store genetic information.

A score above the Lab Reference Range may suggest:
- Gout
- Kidney malfunction/kidney stones
- Hypertension
- Leukemia

- Pregnancy toxemia
- The side effect of diuretic drugs
- Magnesium and B complex deficiency
- Over-consumption of alcohol, desserts, starches and organ meats

It is unusual for an excessively low score to occur but not unusual for a score to be below the Lab Reference Range. Review your score with your doctor if you are concerned.

16. Total Protein

Protein is a diverse and important component of your blood. Your total protein score helps your physician understand your body's metabolic function (the blood's capability for transporting nutrients within your body), as well as your body's overall defensive capability.

Formed primarily in the liver, there are several distinct types of proteins, each with its own function. (These specific proteins are explained next.) Blood proteins are not in the same form as the proteins you eat. Dietary proteins are composed of amino acids, the building blocks of protein. Amino acids are then absorbed into your bloodstream through the upper intestine and carried throughout your body. There are many amino acids, each with its own function. Vegetarians need to be meticulous with their choice of protein foods and should test to double-check their protein levels. Be a cautious vegetarian and be sure your plan is working. Most vegetarians who are not nutrition-aware may be out of balance. Testing can reveal these imbalances and prevent progression to disease states.

Having less than perfect scores for protein can mean you do not eat enough protein in general. Or, you do not eat enough of high quality protein foods making digestion and utilization more difficult. Another reason for less than optimum scores could be consumption of protein foods along with too many carbohydrates. This causes poor digestion and, therefore, poor utilization and absorption.

A score above the Lab Reference Range may suggest:
- Dehydration
- Multiple myeloma (a widespread growth of microscopic plasma cells in organs and bones)

A score below the Lab Reference Range may indicate:
- Excessive protein elimination through kidneys
- Chronic loss of blood
- Insufficient dietary protein or fasting
- Advanced stages of hypertension leading to heart failure
- Hodgkin's disease
- Certain types of degenerative diseases
- Temporary excessive fluid retention
- A weakened immune system due to low intake of protein, as well as imbalance of essential amino acids

17. Albumin

Albumin makes up about 60 percent of the proteins in your blood. Blood proteins like albumin (and globulin, described next) are not the same as the protein in the food you eat, but become amino acids through digestion. These are absorbed through your bloodstream and carried throughout your body.

Albumin helps to maintain the proper pressure of fluids between your vascular system and the surrounding cells. If liquid does seep from one system to the other, albumin soaks it up like a sponge and returns it to its proper place.

You should have an albumin test if:
- You have just experienced heavy blood loss
- You experience bloating and swelling of tissue

A score above the Lab Reference Range may indicate:
- Dehydration
- Stress

A score below the Lab Reference Range may indicate:
- Malnutrition or starvation
- Kidney dysfunction
- Cirrhosis of the liver
- Infections
- Kidney failure
- Gastrointestinal diseases
- Hepatitis
- Maglobulinmia (inability of body to form sufficient antibodies causing chronic leukemia and lymphoma)
- Insufficient intake of complete proteins in the diet

18. Globulin

As indicated, globulin also becomes an amino acid through digestion. Globulins act as the transportation agents for vital nutrients and other components in your blood. Some globulins also act as defense agents within your body.

Globulins can be broken down into alpha and beta globulins. These transport sex hormones, hormones released by the thyroid gland, various forms of copper, iron, cholesterol and other important bloodstream components.

The best-known globulins are gamma globulins, which are composed of a variety of protective antibodies. Natural gamma globulins present in mother's milk protect newborns until they can manufacture their own antibodies.

A score above the Lab Reference Range for gamma globulins may indicate:
- Allergies
- Infections
- Cirrhosis of the liver
- Anemia
- Rheumatoid arthritis
- Some leukemias
- Lupus
- Hodgkin's disease
- Chronic liver disease

- Multiple myeloma (a widespread growth of microscopic plasma cells in organs and bones)

A score below the Lab Reference Range for gamma globulins may indicate:
- Agammaglobulinemia (inability of the body to form sufficient antibodies)
- Kidney disease
- Degenerative diseases
- Lymphoma
- Starvation
- Weak immune system
- Poor protein digestion, absorption and transportation for cell metabolism

19. Albumin/Globulin Ratio

The albumin/globulin ratio is the albumin score divided by the globulin score. For example, if your albumin score is 4.7 and your globulin score is 2.8, then your ratio is 1.68 or 1.7. This is a normal score by most lab standards.

A score above or below the Lab Reference Range may indicate:
- An imbalance of each of the scores
- An imbalance of one of the scores
- Weak immune system due to imbalance of protein utilization or intake
- A vegetarian diet that is not properly balanced for nutritional deficiencies

20. Gallbladder/Bile Enzyme Test (GGTP)

GGTP tests the liver and gallbladder and is used by your doctor to diagnose gallbladder, pancreatic or liver disease. If you have had colon or breast cancer, this test will be very helpful for watching the trend of the results over time. Colon and breast cancer can spread to the liver, gallbladder or pancreas. The objective is to have the lowest possible score.

Consuming alcohol and caffeine as well as recreational use of drugs can affect this score.

A GGTP test helps recovering alcoholics monitor their liver recovery process. They need to heal their livers. Decreasing scores (especially if using the herb milk thistle to help rebuild new tissue) is an indicator of renewed liver health and function.

The pancreas, liver and gallbladder are responsible for producing enzymes and bile to digest foods. If you overload on fats and/or carbohydrates, you may trigger severe abdominal pain caused by poor digestion. Your GGTP score may possibly be elevated.

A score above the Lab Reference Range may suggest:
- Gallbladder disease (very prevalent in women over the age of forty who are overweight)
- Alcoholism, cirrhosis of the liver
- Cancer of the pancreas, liver or gallbladder
- Hyperthyroidism

- Overuse of medications containing acetaminophen (like Tylenol)

A score below the Lab Reference Range must be evaluated in relationship to other tests to determine its significance.

21. Serum Glutamic-Oxaloacetic Transaminase

Serum Glutamic-Oxaloacetic Transaminase, or SGOT, sometimes labeled AST, is an enzyme present in body tissues (heart, liver, kidney, brain, skeletal muscles, spleen and lungs) when proteins are broken down into energy.

SGOT levels, when viewed in combination with other scores, and when the location of the symptoms is taken into account, could help diagnose organ damage. An abnormal elevation of SGOT may indicate a disease affecting any of the tissues mentioned above. However, it does predominatly indicate heart problems.

A score above the Lab Reference Range may suggest:
- Diseases of the kidney, brain, skeletal muscles, spleen, or lungs
- Damage to the heart muscle resulting from a heart attack
- Liver conditions such as viral hepatitis, chemical poisoning, infectious mononucleosis, cirrhosis, obstructive jaundice
- Hormone deficiency
- Chemical toxicity

A score below the Lab Reference Range must be evaluated in relation to other tests to determine its significance.

22. Serum Glutamic-pyruvic Transaminase

Serum Glutamic-pyruvic Transaminase, or SGPT, sometimes called ALT, is an enzyme that helps metabolize protein, a process that takes place primarily in the liver. An increase in SGPT is a warning signal for liver disease.

A score above the Lab Reference may suggest:
- Hepatitis
- Cirrhosis
- Excessive caffeine intake
- Excessive alcohol intake
- Medication overload or incompatibility
- Chemical toxicity (caused by recreational drugs, as well as prescription or excessive over the-counter drug use)

23. Lactic Dehydrogenase (LDH)

Lactic dehydrogenase (LDH) is an enzyme that converts lactic acid to pyruvic acid, which helps metabolize carbohydrates, fats, and amino acids.

LDH is present in most tissues. An elevated LDH level in the blood indicates damage to the heart, kidneys, liver and skeletal tissues. The heart contains proportionately more LDH than other body tissues, and so, high levels usually accompany heart attacks.

High LDH levels also result in liver damage and blood cell disorders. Sometimes further testing for LDH is necessary to pinpoint its origin as it is made up of five separate proteins.

A score above the Lab Reference Range can indicate:
- Tissue damage
- Heart attacks
- Congestive heart failure
- Myocarditis (inflammation of the heart)
- Megaloblastic anemia (B_{12} or folic acid deficiency)
- Certain leukemias
- Liver damage from hepatitis, cirrhosis, and jaundice

False readings may occur if the blood was drawn or handled improperly.

24. Bilirubin (Total and Direct)

Bilirubin is composed mostly of the pigment of red blood cells that have died as a normal part of the constant process of regeneration and renewal in your body.

Bilirubin is a waste product of hemoglobin, the oxygen-carrying red blood cells. It is converted from indirect (non water-soluble) to direct (water-soluble) forms so that it can be eliminated from your body. An elevated level of indirect bilirubin may indicate an excessive rate of red blood cells breaking down caused by certain industrial poisons and insecticides. Or it may be a side-effect of medications. An elevated level of direct bilirubin may also indicate problems with your liver or bile drainage system.

Testing for bilirubin can help identify liver, bile duct or red blood cell disorders. The Comprehensive Panel, offered by YFH, includes the test for the total bilirubin and the direct bilirubin. You can determine your indirect bilirubin by subtracting the direct bilirubin score from the total bilirubin score. This equals the indirect bilirubin score, or TB minus DB equals IB.

A score above the Lab Reference Range for total bilirubin may indicate:
- An excess of alcohol or caffeine intake
- Cancer
- Degenerative disease
- A previous bout of a disease of the liver such as hepatitis or cirrhosis
- An overuse of medications or drugs

A score above the Lab Reference Range for direct bilirubin may indicate:
- Gallstones
- Tumors
- Infection or Inflammation

A score below the Lab Reference Range must be evaluated in relation to other tests to determine its significance.

25. White Blood Cells (WBC)

White blood cells are the Marine Corps of the body; the few, the proud, the fighters. The white blood cells are our first-line of defense against infection. Compared to the number of red blood cells in our bodies, there are very few white blood cells.

White blood cells are specialized, too. Each type has a specific function for fighting disease. Because of these differences, doctors will order a differential count to pinpoint which white blood cells are responsible for the infection. Elevations outside of the Lab Reference Range of the specific WBCs show that you are overworking your immune system. Remember to check your serum zinc level. Zinc is usually destroyed when your immune system is overworked.

A score above the Lab Reference Range may suggest:
- Bacterial infection
- Appendicitis
- Inflammatory condition
- Leukemia
- Hemolytic anemia in newborns
- Normal pregnancy
- Excessive and/or strenuous exercise
- Anxiety or emotional stress

A score below the Lab Reference Range may suggest:
- Viral infection
- Radiation exposure
- Anti-rejection therapy in organ transplant recipients
- Side effects of some anti-cancer therapies
- Rheumatoid arthritis
- Cirrhosis of the liver
- Lupus erythematosis, which affects the skin only

26. Red Blood Count (RBC)

Red blood cells (RBCs) transport oxygen from your lungs throughout your body. It takes approximately six days for a red blood cell to be manufactured in the bone marrow and released. Once in the bloodstream, the cell functions for 100-120 days and then dies and is replaced. Over the period of a year, all the red blood cells in your body are replaced completely about three times.

Polycythemia is the result of overproduction of red blood cells. However, this is not always bad. If you live at a high altitude, your body produces more red blood cells because you need more oxygen in the thinner air

YFH has different optimum RBC score suggestions for people of different height, weight, gender, age, etc. It is not "one-size-fits-all," but rather what has proven optimum for our clients over the years.

A score above the Lab Reference Range may suggest:
- Symptoms of polycythemia
- Poor circulation (with symptoms such as cold extremities, poor color to nails)
- High blood pressure (hypertension)
- Clotting within the blood vessels
- Stroke, emphysema or congenital heart disease
- Dehydration

A score below the Lab Reference Range may suggest:
- Folic acid and/or B_{12} deficiencies
- Aplastic anemia, occurs when bone marrow tissue is

destroyed by exposure to chemicals such as benzene, insecticides and various anti-cancer drugs, plus some prescription drugs

- Hemolytic anemia (body produces antibodies that destroy its own red blood cells); occurs in leukemia, certain kinds of malignant tumors, syphilis, hepatitis, lupus, arthritis, kidney and degenerative diseases

27. Hemoglobin (HGB)

Hemoglobin is the part of your red blood cell that carries oxygen from your lungs to the cells of your body. Hemoglobin production takes place in the bone marrow as a part of the manufacturing of red blood cells.

Reasons for testing hemoglobin level include:
- Fatigue
- Exposure to lead
- Sickle cell anemia
- Low iron level in blood
- Heavy menstrual periods or excessive loss of blood
- Low iron intake

Identifying a decreasing trend in hemoglobin that eventually falls below the Lab Reference Range may lead to early cancer detection as based on clients' results.

A score above the Lab Reference Range may indicate:
- Excessive testosterone production (can occur in males or females)
- Excessive red blood cell production

A score below the Lab Reference Range may suggest:
- Anemia

YFH believes, based on the clinical data from its clients, that anemia can be due to an iron deficiency or B-vitamin deficiency, especially a deficiency in folic acid and B_{12}.

28. Hematocrit (HCT)

Hematocrit (HCT) is a blood test named after the special capillary tube in which the test is done. The HCT measures the portion of blood made up of red blood cells by spinning the blood in a capillary tube with a centrifuge. A centrifuge is a machine that spins the blood test tube at extremely high speeds in order to the separate serum from the whole cells of the blood.

A score above the Lab Reference Range may suggest:
- Dehydration, often caused by diarrhea and vomiting
- Polycythemia (an increased concentration of red blood cells that can lead to stroke)

A score below the Lab Reference Range may suggest:
- Anemia

29. Platelets

Platelets are the glue of the blood. When you cut or bruise yourself, platelets clump together and seal breaks in even the tiniest blood vessels. They form a temporary plug until a more permanent clot can be formed. In the case of a bruise, the platelets glue the break in the capillary walls to stop the loss of blood into the tissues.

Anticoagulant drugs (used to reduce the likelihood of heart attacks) prevent this process, and therefore, random bruising occurs when tissue is damaged.

The nutrient eicosapentaenoic acid (EPA—an omega 3 fatty acid composed of fish oil) is very valuable in preventing blood clots. It makes the platelets slippery to prevent clot formation, and promotes ease of movement of the platelets inside the blood vessel. However, it does not prevent the normal clotting mechanism from working should you cut yourself. Diabetics usually have thick blood and are prone to clots. EPA may be helpful but consult your doctor or health professional before taking it in supplemental form. Be sure to do the Omega 3 Profile+ test to determine the amount of EPA fish oil you may need.

A score above the Lab Reference Range may suggest:
- Blood loss due to hemorrhage
- A breakdown of red blood cells
- Inflammatory diseases (arthritis, fibromyalgia)
- Certain malignancies
- Polycythemia vera (increased RBC concentration)

A score below the Lab Reference Range may suggest:
- Poor platelet production as found in anemia related to folic acid deficiencies
- Damage to bone marrow tissue, as in aplastic anemia

- Platelets destroyed through the antibody defense mechanism

30. Mean Corpuscular Volume (MCV)

One of three "mean" tests, MCV helps distinguish several kinds of anemia and thus determines the most appropriate kind of treatment. See the next two tests, MCH and MCHC for the other two "means" tests.

MCV refers to the relative volume of each red blood cell or its average size. This test helps determine the size and oxygen-carrying capacity of individual red blood cells. If MCV is not at its optimum level, you may feel very tired even if you have enough red blood cells because the cells are not healthy enough to carry oxygen properly. Without oxygen, you feel exhausted. You can exercise and deep breathe regularly, but if the oxygen-carrying ability is not at its peak you will still feel tired.

To understand more about this test, you must first read about the MCHC test in this section. The two tests are used together to determine different types of anemias that could be present.

A score above the Lab Reference Range may indicate:
- Anemia due to a deficiency of folic acid during pregnancy
- Pernicious anemia (vitamin B_{12} deficiency)

A score on the upper end of the reference range (7100) usually indicates macrocytosis (large red blood cells that may be large enough to carry Hgb-O_2 [hemoglobin-oxygen] but may not be Hgb [hemoglobin] filled enough). See MCH and MCHC scores to determine this.

A score below the Lab Reference Range may indicate:
- Iron deficiency anemia
- Bleeding in the digestive tract or urinary tract
- Excessive menstrual bleeding

A score on the lower end of the reference range (80 or below) usually indicates microcytosis (small red blood cells that are not large enough to carry much oxygen).

31. Mean Corpuscular Hemoglobin (MCH)

MCH is the second of the three "means." Although we refer to MCH as a test, it is actually a calculation based on two other tests. To calculate MCH, divide the hemoglobin score by the number of red blood cells and multiply by ten.

It is important to keep a watchful eye on your MCH score in combination with your RBC and hemoglobin scores. Our observation shows that our clients had a serious decline in their MCH, RBC and hemoglobin levels prior to a diagnosis of cancer. Achieving optimum scores for these three components is critical to properly oxygenate your tissues, which YFH believes may reduce risk of cancer.

A score above the Lab Reference Range may indicate:
- Anemia
- Deficiency of vitamins B_{12} and folic acid

- Iron deficiency
- Exhaustion
- Weight gain
- Pregnancy

32. Mean Corpuscular Hemoglobin Concentration (MCHC)

The third "mean" is MCHC. This test measures the relative volume of hemoglobin in the average red blood cell—that is, the portion of each red blood cell that is hemoglobin.

MCHC and MCV together are used to identify types of anemia.

A MCV and MCHC score that is 30 percent higher than the Lab Reference Range may indicate:
- Pernicious anemia (lack of vitamin B_{12})

YFH clinical data suggest that an increase of vitamin B_{12} in foods and supplements enhance these scores.

MCHC and MCV scores below the Lab Reference Range may indicate iron deficiency anemia caused by:
- Chronic digestive disorders (stomach or intestinal), urinary bleeding or surgery
- Excessive menstruation (exhausting iron reserves)
- Repeated pregnancies (increased demand for hemoglobin and RBCs that result in folic acid deficiency)
- Anemias caused by genetic abnormalities

An MCV score that is within the Lab Reference Range in combination with an MCHC Lab Reference score greater than 30 percent plus a low Lab Reference hemoglobin and/or red blood cell count may indicate these problems:

- Hemolytic anemia (body produces antibodies to destroy red blood cells)
- Hemophilia (genetic disease causing inability for blood to clot)
- Sickle cell anemia (red blood cells are abnormal and crescent-shaped, causing reduced oxygen supplies, which predominantly affect people of African descent)
- Aplastic anemia (damage to bone marrow tissue)
- Anemias associated with infections, malignancies (cancer) and kidney diseases

33. Red Cell Distribution Width (RDW)

This test is done to help determine the size of a red blood cell or red corpuscle. RDW must be within particular limits to properly carry oxygen. When the result is at the highest end of the Lab Reference Range, you usually feel somewhat tired and anemic because the cells are unable to oxygenate tissue properly.

Consider ordering an RDW test if:
- Your RBC count is consistently within the Lab Reference Range but you are more tired than usual
- You are on cancer drugs that may alter the health of your red blood cells

To fully understand the meaning of the RDW score, one must evaluate the following scores in relation to one another: RBC, hemoglobin, HCT, MCV, MCH, MCHC, iron, and ferritin. If an RDW score is outside the Lab Reference Range, one or more of these scores will not be optimum as well. Once again, this illustrates the need to do many tests since several are interrelated.

A score above the Lab Reference Range may indicate:
- Anemia
- Low level or poor utilization of iron
- Anisocytosis, a variation in size of red blood cells

A score below the Lab Reference Range may indicate:
- Anemia
- Destruction of red blood cells

34. Manual RBC Morphology

Manual red blood cell morphology tests for types of anemia including iron and B vitamin deficiencies, which can result in poor oxygenation of tissue. Generally, a less expensive test called an automated RBC morphology is performed. A machine with pre-set levels analyzes the test for illness and reports anything abnormal. YFH insists that a skilled technician personally views the specimen through a microscope and interprets the results. By doing a manual red blood cell morphology test in addition to the automated test, early signs of anemia can be noted. With the automated test alone, abnormalities are often not noticed until they become severe.

The manual red blood cell morphology test is very valuable. Many of our clients complain of fatigue, yet their doctors' reports show that all their tests are "normal." Often their fatigue comes from a lack of B vitamins and iron. The low levels of B vitamins and/or iron interfere with the red blood cells' ability to properly carry oxygen to cells and thus the feeling of fatigue. Based on our clients' results over the last twenty-six years, YFH believes that this test is instrumental in helping to catch cancer early.

RBC Morphology Abnormalities

Anisocytosis: Variation in size of RBCs
Poikilocytosis: Variation in shape of RBCs
Microcytosis: Smaller than normal RBCs, less than 7 microns in diameter
Macrocytosis: Larger than normal RBCs, greater than 10 microns in diameter
Hypochromasia: RBCs that are pale pink in color due to insufficient hemoglobin
Polychromasia: RBCs that are grayish blue in color due to immaturity of cells
Ovalocytes: RBCs that are oval in shape
Elliptocytes: RBCs that are elliptical in shape
Target Cells: RBCs that are shaped like a target with a bull's eye (often due to anemia or if spleen is removed)

35. Total Cholesterol

The truth about cholesterol is much more complex than the popular reputation as an indicator of heart disease. It is not in your best health interest to cut all cholesterol from your diet. Extremely low levels can be just as unhealthful as extremely high levels.

Cholesterol is essential to life. Cholesterol:
- Makes possible the passage of vital substances through cell walls
- Keeps us from becoming waterlogged when we bathe
- Is essential for hormones involved in sex drive and reproduction
- Keeps us from becoming salt-depleted in hot climates

Your body (mainly your liver) manufactures 70 percent of the total cholesterol found in your liver, skin, adrenal glands, intestines, testes and ovaries. The remaining 30 percent of your body's cholesterol comes from the foods you eat.

A score of 250 is not problematic if your HDL (good cholesterol) is 125. The cholesterol/HDL ratio would then be 2.0, which is very good. Discuss this with your doctor, but do not panic if your cholesterol score is 200 or higher. If your LDL (bad cholesterol) is low and HDL is high then the ratios are low as well. You may be just fine. Remember: never accept a total cholesterol score as important unless you see the other scores. (HDL, LDL, and the cholesterol/HDL ratio).

A score above the Lab Reference Range may indicate:
- No problem if the HDL is very high and LDL is low
- Biliary cirrhosis of the liver/bile duct blockage
- Cushing's syndrome (over-activity of adrenal cortex)
- Uncontrolled sugar diabetes
- Increased plaque formation in blood vessels

A score below the Lab Reference Range may indicate:

- Stress
- Poor intestinal absorption
- Deficiency of essential fatty acids

36. High-Density Lipoprotein (HDL)

One of the possible answers to the mystery of the connection between cholesterol and heart disease appears to be the way cholesterol combines with protein and is carried in the blood.

A high proportion of the "good" cholesterol, high-density lipoprotein or HDL, is an indication that you may have a much lower risk for a heart attack. But for certainty, do the VAP test.

A good way to increase the HDL proportion in your blood is through exercise. Physically active people have a higher proportion of this good cholesterol in relation to their total cholesterol than do more sedentary people.

An elevated HDL reading is not the only factor involved in avoiding heart attacks. Other factors include:
- Weight
- Stress levels
- Smoking habits
- Blood pressure
- Family health history
- Elimination (good elimination of bowels helps to keep cholesterol levels at normal range)
- Fiber and water intake (assists elimination)
- Homocysteine levels

A score below the normal Lab Reference Range indicates:
- Not enough physical activity
- Too many cholesterol-rich foods in your diet
- Increased risk of coronary heart disease
- Increased plaque deposits on blood vessel walls

37. Cholesterol/HDL Ratio

We all know people who watch their diets carefully for cholesterol and fat and yet have heart attacks. We know others who seem to eat whatever they want and have no heart problems. And we know that 75 percent of heart attacks happen to people whose cholesterol levels are in the normal range.

Part of the reason for these confusing statistics appears to be the way cholesterol combines with proteins and is transported in your blood. HDL attaches itself to high-density lipoprotein. The higher the proportion of HDL in your blood, the less the risk of having heart attacks. See the VAP test for more details about HDL.

The best way to raise the level of HDL in your blood is to increase your activity. Joggers and physically active people usually register a high HDL level in proportion to the total cholesterol in the blood. You may raise your HDL level about 25 percent by exercising vigorously for thirty minutes, at least four times per week.

Diet also plays an important part in the total cholesterol/ HDL ratio. All cholesterol rich foods are not bad for you.

Foods that are high in carbohydrates and high on the glycemic index are more likely to cause an imbalance.

38. Low-Density Lipoprotein (LDL)

Low-density lipoprotein, or LDL, like HDL, combines with proteins and is carried in the blood. However, this is the "bad" cholesterol, that deposits plaque on your artery walls. Plaque clogs your arteries and frequently leads to atherosclerosis (plaque build-up on vessel walls, reducing the opening through which blood can flow) and to heart attacks. Plaque deposits can begin at birth. The trick is to slow the process with the help of diet and exercise. Those who learn about the right diet, supplements and exercise rarely require drugs to lower cholesterol.

Some people believe that they have a high LDL level because of family history and that the high score is normal for them. I encourage people to ask their doctors to do a Doppler test (a non-invasive test) to determine how much plaque is on the vessel walls. Pay for this test even if your insurance will not. Have one done yearly and track your results. Do the VAP blood test to determine your genetic pattern.

Studies indicate that other dietary factors, such as high levels of sugar, may determine whether cholesterol remains in the blood in excess levels.

A score above the Lab Reference Range may indicate:
- Not enough physical activity
- Possible genetic influence, indicating the need to

strictly follow diet and exercise recommendations
- A diet high in sugar and junk foods
- Increased risk of coronary heart disease
- Consumption of processed fats

39. Triglycerides

Look in the mirror and you might see triglycerides. These lipids are responsible for midriff bulge, jowls, and/or fatty deposits in thighs and buttocks. That's because triglycerides are stored in special cells called adipose tissue, which is concentrated in these areas.

Triglycerides are made in the liver from excess carbohydrates, especially sugar and alcohol. They are an important source of energy for your body and have the highest caloric value per weight of any body material.

Although the triglycerides deposited in adipose tissue may be unattractive, they are not the real culprits leading to heart disease. Triglycerides in the bloodstream, however, are a strong indicator of possible coronary disease. Shortly after you consume triglycerides, they form chylomicrons, which are droplets of fat used by the body for energy. If you consume more triglycerides than your body needs for energy, they will be stored as fat.

If the body cannot remove the chylomicrons, they slow blood circulation. Eventually, the chylomicrons are deposited on the arterial walls and form plaque, which increases the risk of heart attacks and cardiovascular disease.

A triglyceride score above the Lab Reference Range may indicate:
- Excess fats, sugars or alcohol in the diet
- Overproduction of triglycerides in the liver
- Severe deficiency of thyroid hormones (be sure to test Free T4, Thyroid Uptake, and TSH)
- A need for a high protein diet devoid of high glycemic and high carbohydrate food
- Bile duct dysfunction

A score below the Lab Reference Range must be evaluated relative to other tests to determine its significance.

40. TG/HDL Ratio

The ratio between your triglycerides (TG) and your HDL cholesterol level gives you more information about the type of cholesterol that is in your blood. Dividing your triglycerides by your HDL score will give you this ratio.

Cholesterol has conventionally been divided into two groups-the "bad" LDL and the "good" HDL. New research has shown us that there are fluffy "good/protective" and dense "non-protective" cholesterol within both the HDL and LDL categories.

If your score for the TG/HDL ratio is less than 1.5, the "bad" LDL cholesterol may be primarily made of the large fluffy particles that do not cause as much harm as the denser non-protective ones that are associated with plaque deposits and increase the risk of heart disease. However, if your ratio is above 1.5, your LDL cholesterol is primarily made of the small dense particles that can accelerate the development of arteriosclerosis, or plaque, *regardless* of your total cholesterol levels.

In an unceasing search for more precise information to help guide you to wellness, YFH does an expanded cholesterol test that identifies your genetic pattern to see if you are pre-disposed to high cholesterol levels and whether you have the dense or fluffy cholesterol. This new expanded cholesterol test is explained in exciting detail under the VAP test. Please see the reference section for more research supporting these concepts.

41. Neutrophils

Segmented neutrophils make up more than half of the white blood cells in the body. Produced in the bone marrow, they enter the body's tissues within twenty-four hours.

If there is an infection somewhere in your body, neutrophils move in large numbers to that site and destroy the bacteria by engulfing them. If no infection exists, the neutrophils self-destruct.

A score above the Lab Reference Range may indicate:
- Bacterial infections
- Acute appendicitis
- Leukemia
- Physiological changes resulting from fear, anger or exposure to extreme heat or cold
- Excessive or severe exercise

- Certain drugs (such as digitalis)
- Poisons

A score below the Lab Reference Range may indicate:
- The onset of infections
- Certain prescription drugs (like drugs for gout and cancer)
- Excess alcohol intake
- A very weak immune system

42. Eosinophils

Like other white blood cells, eosinophils are manufactured in the bone marrow. In addition to protecting the lungs, skin and gastrointestinal tract, they help fight against allergic reactions.

When you have an allergic reaction, your body reacts by overproducing antibodies. Eosinophils can digest the antigen that produces the antibodies.

A score above the Lab Reference Range may suggest:
- Allergic reaction or eczema
- Bronchial asthma
- Hay fever
- Skin reactions to medication
- Scarlet fever
- Parasitic infection of the intestinal tract
- Eosinophilic leukemia

Because a perfect score is zero, there is no advice for being below the Lab Reference Range.

43. Lymphocytes

Lymphocytes are manufactured in the spleen, lymph nodes and intestinal-related lymph tissue. Lymphocytes produce neutralizing antibodies against viral disease.

Because of their antibody-producing capability, lymphocytes play a major role in organ transplants and skin grafts. They can cause organs/grafts to be rejected.

Some lymphocytes live for months and even years in the bloodstream. Because of this, they sometimes cause problems in delayed hypersensitivity. You might not have a reaction to a wasp sting if you get stung a first time, but these lymphocytes will be ready the next time. They will remember the venom as foreign matter. Lymphocytes may overproduce by suddenly releasing histamines and cause a fatal reaction.

Short-lived lymphocytes form antibodies against invading viruses. They do their job and then disappear within a few days.

A score above the Lab Reference Range may indicate:
- Common cold or flu
- Whooping cough
- German measles
- Infectious mononucleosis

A score below the Lab Reference Range may indicate:
- Immune system deficiencies

- Increased levels of ACTH (pituitary hormone) due to stress
- Hodgkin's disease
- Blocked lymphatic system drainage
- Anti-cancer drug therapy
- Anti-rejection therapy

44. Monocytes

Monocytes fight infection in your body.

The largest cells in your blood, monocytes begin their existence in your bone marrow and migrate into your bloodstream. They stay in your bloodstream for about three days, and prepare themselves for battle against infection in the body's tissues.

Like super heroes, monocytes transform into macrophages ready for battle once they enter the tissues. In this new form, they engulf and digest foreign particles as well as the damaged body cells that caused the reaction.

Monocytes can also fight bacteria, pollens and viruses. They can help reduce swelling by ingesting stagnant fluids in inflamed tissues as well.

A score above the Lab Reference Range may suggest:
- Recovery from acute infection including the common cold and flu
- Connective tissue disorders
- Colitis
- Inflammatory disease

- Hodgkin's disease
- Early indication of leukemia

A score below the Lab Reference Range must be evaluated in relation to other tests to determine its significance.

45. Basophils

Basophils are similar in function to eosinophils and neutrophils. They protect body tissues. And they, too, are manufactured in the bone marrow.

Basophils are responsible for histamine (allergic type) reactions, especially in deep tissues like the intestines and liver. If the intestine is under attack, you will usually see an increase in these cells. Additional research as to the function of these cells is ongoing.

Although basophils are white blood cells, they have a deep purple color, which make them easy to see on blood smears in laboratory tests.

An increase in basophils may indicate:
- Allergic reactions
- Polycythemia vera - an excess of red blood cells and total blood volume
- Chronic granulocytic leukemia - an abnormal growth of white blood cells that have granules found in blood forming organs
- An irritation of the intestines or liver as may occur when you have a virus
- Hemolytic anemia (breakdown of RBCs)

Because a perfect score is zero, there is no advice for being below the Lab Reference Range.

46. Bands

Band cells are immature neutrophils. Confined to the bone marrow, their purpose is to develop into mature neutrophils. However, in the case of acute infections, they may be prematurely released to help fight the invading bacteria.

You need to strengthen your immune system if you have a positive band test result. The goal is to have zero bands. While it is good that your body can make bands, it is a sign that you are stressing your immune system. YFH suggests retesting monthly if your score is higher than one. It is not necessary to retest if your doctor tells you not to worry, or if you know you had an illness at the time you tested and you had not fully recovered. However, if you are unsure why your score is not zero, it is best to retest.

A score above the Lab Reference Range may indicate:
- High demand for neutrophils
- Unexplained increase in bone marrow production of white blood cells (check with your doctor immediately)
- Weakened immune system

Because a perfect score is zero, there is no advice for being below the Lab Reference Range.

47. Atypical Lymphocytes

Atypical white blood cells with irregular shape and size are derived from lymph tissue and are abnormal. Zero is the desired score at all times. If you have these cells, this may indicate the presence of infection. Your lymph nodes work very hard when you are sick. The presence of atypical lymphocytes usually suggests that your immune system is severely taxed.

A score above the Lab Reference Range may suggest:
- Severe infection or various viral infections
- Cancer (skin, lymph system, etc.)
- Weakened immune system
- Infectious mononucleosis

Because a perfect score is zero, there is no advice for being below the Lab Reference Range.

48. Prostatic Specific Antigen (PSA)

Sometimes known as the male Pap test, this test is used to screen for prostate cancer. Prostatic specific antigen (PSA) is a protease enzyme that is produced by the epithelial cells of prostatic tissue. It is present in high combinations in seminal fluid.

A normal level of serum PSA is not a guarantee that you are cancer-free. And an elevated level may not always indicate cancer, since prostate massage, prostate examination or the drug clofibrate may cause an elevated reading. But without these possibilities, an elevated reading is an indication that prostate cancer may be present.

It is especially important to have a benchmark score for this test before age 55 (the customary age to start testing) because the best indication of prostate cancer is the sudden increasing trend of this score. For example, if your score is always in a range of 2 to 2.8 and it suddenly jumps to 4.2, this increase is very significant. Because the score is so close to normal, according to the Lab Reference Range, it may be ignored. That's why the comparison between tests is so important. To learn more about how tracking your trend can be valuable, read about Harold F. Miller's experience in our case study section.

A score above the Lab Reference Range may indicate:
- Prostatitis (infected prostate)
- Prostate cancer
- Benign enlarged prostate

49. Total Prostatic Specific Antigen and Free % Prostatic Specific Antigen (PSA II)

PSA II is made up of two tests: the Total PSA and the Free % PSA. It is imperative when comparing scores to use the same methodology each time and the same lab equipment for performing both tests. The cost is slightly more because this test is so highly specialized. A second analysis must be done whenever a Free % PSA is done. The lowest possible Total PSA, score preferably below 1.0, in combination with a score that is higher than 25% Free PSA score, preferably 100%, is the goal.

Why should you have a PSA II test done instead of a Total PSA test? After age forty, as the risk of developing prostate cancer increases, a more complete analysis is necessary. The PSA II is more accurate and will give you greater peace of mind. If your scores for a Total PSA have been rising (although still within the reference range) you should have the more thorough test done to see if there is a problem. Do not trust that higher scores outside the lab normal reference range are expected just because you are older. By ordering the PSA II, you can determine whether the prostate is enlarging with age or if cancer is developing. The power of this test is the ability to detect the very beginning of a problem in time to make corrections and lower the scores before you have cancer.

A score above the Lab Reference Range for both scores may indicate:
- Cancer of the prostate

50. CA 125

The CA 125 test is a female cancer screen. It tests for ovarian and primary peritoneal cancer. We feel that this test should be done for virtually every woman. It provides a benchmark score that is invaluable. This test should not be done when pregnant or during menstruation.

The usual lab normal reference range is between 0 and 20 if tested on the new Immulite 2000 machine. If your score is consistently around 5 to 10, and suddenly jumps to 21, this could be significant. The score of 21 is so close to normal that your doctor may consider this to be okay. Especially if your doctor did not have your blood test history. But if you have repeated this test over time and tracked your results, you can share this blood test history information with your doctor. The comparative scores for this test, like the PSA test for men, are more important than one isolated score. Insurance companies typically cover the cost of this test only if it is used to detect recurrence of cancer.

If your score is higher than 20, you should see your doctor immediately and let him/her decide its significance. It may only mean that you have an ovarian cyst or a benign fibroid tumor, but it should be checked. Additional tests may be needed. If you have elevated results for the CA 125 test, extra tests may be able to be justified for coverage by your insurance company.

A score above the Lab Reference Range may indicate:
* Ovarian or primary peritoneal cancer
* Fibroid or ovarian tumor

Please note that a lab normal reference range of 0 to 35 usually indicates that different equipment other than the Immulite 2000 machine was used. The scores from the two machines should not be compared.

51. Carcinoembryonic Antigen (CEA)

The CEA serum blood test remains the best tumor marker available as a one-test, one-score indicator of colon cancer as well as seven other types of cancer. Although it has limitations, the CEA test is still the most accurate indicator of impending disease. It can detect the presence of cancer from three to thirty-six months before physical symptoms develop. This allows time to make diet corrections, to supplement, to exercise and to follow stress reduction programs while the immune system is still responsive. These actions may cure the problem before it becomes a disease. It is imperative to do a comprehensive blood test, which includes a serum zinc test and an alkaline phosphatase, at the same time as the CEA. This provides sufficient data to interpret the CEA test results appropriately. Without having the additional tests, it would be apparent that there is a problem but it would be difficult to determine which one of your body systems is being affected.

Types of cancer that can be detected by the CEA test include lung, bone, breast, liver, pancreatic, thyroid and stomach to colon. This is an opportunity to find these diseases early enough so that you can control the disease.

How does the test work? You compare your CEA scores each time you test. Your body is giving you a chance to make corrections before you feel sick. Observe your symptoms each time you test. Negative symptoms may correlate to negative test changes. Recording your symptoms may help your doctor find the reason for future, higher elevations. Scores between 10 and 20 are much more likely to indicate cancer. Test results above the Lab Reference Range should be shared with your doctor. Let him/her decide their significance. Tests that may be needed to help confirm disease should be covered by insurance or Medicare.

A score above the Lab Reference Range may indicate:
- Possible cancer of lung, bone, thyroid, breast, liver, pancreas, intestinal (stomach to colon)

52. CA 15-3

The CA 15-3 test in combination with the CEA test is one of the best examples of preventive versus symptom driven blood testing. This test is rarely ordered unless there are symptoms of breast cancer, such as a lump or discharge. It is usually ordered for women who have already been diagnosed with breast cancer as a tool to monitor the progress of the disease. YFH has found that some women have breast cancer even when their scores are within the normal lab reference range. Testing the CA 15-3 in combination with the CEA, and following these tests over time will allow an accurate trend to become evident. It is an excellent alert to the early development of breast cancer. The earlier a disease is detected, even though no symptoms may be present, the more effective treatment can be. The sudden jump in scores for *one* of these tests may suggest an irregularity, but a sudden jump in *both* can act as an alarm for breast cancer and should be discussed with your doctor immediately.

A score above the Lab Reference Range indicates:
- Initial breast cancer
- Recurrence of breast cancer

A score below the Lab Reference Range indicates:
- To be meaningful, should be compared to CEA trend and the CA-15-3 trend coupled with a physical exam by your doctor and possible mammogram and/or ultrasound tests

Note that most labs use a reference range that is lower for young women and allows a higher reference range for older women, as they tend to have more cysts that can trigger a higher normal score. Again, it is the trend that helps this test be effective for prevention. Read Judy Flickinger's story in the case study section to see how this saved her life.

53. CA 19-9

CA 19-9 is an exciting new test that is useful to both men and women. It is being used to monitor gastrointestinal and liver cancers; head, neck and gynecological tumors; predict the reoccurrence of stomach, pancreatic and colorectal cancer; as well as liver and gallbladder tumors with varying degrees of accuracy. Although valuable in all these areas, it is most accurate in confirming pancreatic cancer which accounts for 80% of its usage.

When this test is done in combination with the CEA test, an even more complete evaluation can be made. Tracking these tests over time, if done by the same equipment and laboratory, will allow a trend to become evident. If a sudden elevation occurs for these scores, this acts as an alert even if they are still within the normal range. This does not necessarily mean you have cancer, but a retest within a few months is in order to be sure that your levels return to your

Personal Normal. If a sudden "alert" occurs, be sure to bring this to the attention of your doctor.

A score above the Lab Reference Range indicates:
- The need for future testing and evaluation to detect possible pancreatic or stomach disease, head and neck tumors, liver, gallbladder and colorectal disease especially if the CEA is also elevated

A score below the Lab Reference Range indicates:
- A score below the Lab Reference Range is generally considered normal. However, again watch for the sudden jump in the CA-19-9 and/or the CEA scores as an indicator of possible impending disease

54. T3 Uptake

The T3 Uptake is confusing because one thinks it is a T3 test. It is not. It is simply a way to find out if your thyroid has enough tyrosine or casein. If it does not, your thyroid may not be able to do its job properly. Many individuals are on milk-free and low-salt diets, which may affect their thyroid gland if they do not supplement with enough iodine and casein. Milk and table salt are the usual sources of these nutrients. Cheese and seaweed are other possible sources. If you cannot eat any dairy products, you may need a protein supplement made from casein in order to balance this important protein.

A score above the Lab Reference Range may indicate:
- An overactive thyroid
- Sudden weight loss
- Nervousness and sleep problems

A score below the Lab Reference Range may indicate:
- An underactive thyroid
- A lack of sufficient tyrosine (a protein amino acid)
- Weight gain
- Exhaustion, lack of motivation, memory loss

55. Thyroxine (T4)

Total T4 or thyroxine (T4) is a thyroid gland hormone that has four molecules of iodine, thus the name T4. The thyroid gland uses traces of iodine to combine with the amino acid tyrosine to create this molecule. If you are low in tyrosine or protein foods that supply tyrosine (like casein), or if you are low in iodine, you may be prone to an imbalance of your thyroid gland. It is best to discover the signs of this imbalance early, before thyroid activity has either increased or slowed down beyond optimum levels.

Tracking your Thyroid Panel II and your Free T4 numbers is essential to see thyroid changes early and to react to them with dietary improvements. Remember, just because you are eating foods that are balanced and healthy does not mean you are assimilating or fully utilizing these foods. Exercise levels, stress levels, changing calorie needs (as with a nursing mother or pregnancy) require different amounts of nutrients. You need to adjust your foods and supplements accordingly.

Be sure to check your thyroid gland for nodules at least weekly. It is located in the front part of the neck. Have your doctor point out the location at your next exam. If you have an unexplained cough or irritation in your throat or you feel an enlargement or lump, please see your doctor.

A score above the Lab Reference Range may indicate:
- Hyperthyroidism

A score below the Lab Reference Range may indicate:
- Hypothyroidism

56. T7 Free Thyroxine Index

The T7 Index is used to calculate Free T4, one of the two active thyroid hormones in your bloodstream. (The Free T4 test is explained on the next page). This hormone and its sibling, Free T3, are necessary for the delicate and complex process of making your body operate at its proper metabolic rate, and controlling your memory . Our clinical research suggests that early detection of reduced T7 levels help correct body weight imbalances before they become serious problems.

The T7 Index is a calculated Free T4 score and is not as accurate as a machine-run Free T4 test. However, the Free T4 test is expensive and many insurance programs will not cover the cost. The T7, or index test, is included in most thyroid panels. YFH believes that ordering all five thyroid tests is important for a complete picture of the health of your thyroid.

A score above the Lab Reference Range may indicate:
- Hyperthyroidism (symptoms include: cold extremities,

fitful sleep, memory loss, nervous and jumpy feelings, sudden weight loss)

A score below the Lab Reference Range may indicate:
- Hypothyroidism
- Weight gain
- Mental confusion

57. Free T4

Free T4 gets its name because it is the thyroid hormone that frees itself from protein and goes to the area of the body where it is needed. It has four iodine molecules attached to the thyroxine hormone and helps you metabolize your foods. Free T4 is an expensive thyroid test and is not often ordered. It is, however, the best single measurement of thyroid function. YFH includes it in our available tests. It is important to note that iodine and the amino acid, tyrosine, which comes from milk or cheese, are important to include in your diet if you want a well-nourished thyroid gland.

A score above the Lab Reference Range may indicate hyperthyroidism, sometimes called Graves' disease. Symptoms of hyperthyroidism include:
- Jumpiness, nervousness or hand tremors
- Increased perspiration
- Heart palpitations
- Fitful sleep
- Hair loss or changes in softness or sheen
- Sudden weight loss

A score below the Lab Reference Range may indicate hypothyroidism.

Symptoms include:

- Sluggish behavior
- Little or no energy, feeling run down
- Overweight (weight gain may creep up on you)
- Fitful sleep
- Hair loss or changes in softness or sheen

58. Thyroid Stimulating Hormone (TSH)

If you think of your thyroid gland as a furnace, thyroid-stimulating hormone (TSH) is the thermostat that turns the furnace on and off as needed. Thyroid hormones T3 and T4 make up the "fuel" of your furnace. For optimum function of the thyroid gland, a sufficient amount of T3 and T4 hormones need to be produced so they are ready to be released when called for by the TSH. The pituitary gland regulates the release of TSH, which then tells the thyroid gland to release the T3s and T4s as needed. Therefore, when trying to nutritionally balance the thyroid gland, it is also necessary to take into account the needs of the pituitary gland.

YFH data suggests that an imbalance in T3, T4, or TSH causes problems, even if the measurements are within the Lab Reference Range. If you notice fluctuations in your thyroid scores and correct them early on, you may ward off abnormal weight gain, weight loss, lack of energy or memory loss before more serious symptoms develop.

It is inaccurate to assume your thyroid gland needs a boost only on the basis of symptoms. You should be tested and get a benchmark score when your weight is excellent and energy level high. If this is not possible, get tested now and evaluate your symptom changes over the last few years. See if your score gets better with dietary and exercise changes that improve this gland's function while you are still considered normal and do not need medication. Be sure to do the Omega 3 Profile+ test to evaluate your essential fatty acid levels for proper thyroid balance.

A score above the Lab Reference Range may suggest hypothyroidism. Indicators of hypothyroidism are:
- Sluggish behavior, feeling run down, lack of energy
- Gradual unexplained weight gain (no change in eating habits or exercise, yet gaining weight)
- Possible changes in hair loss or hair brittleness
- Change in sleep habits

A score below the Lab Reference Range may suggest hyperthyroidism. Symptoms include:
- Jumpiness and nervousness/change in sleep habits
- Increased perspiration
- Hand tremors/heart palpitations

59. Progesterone

Progesterone is a steroid hormone that plays an important role in preparing the uterus for and maintaining pregnancy. The ovaries and placenta are major production sites for progesterone, but a small amount is also made by the adrenal cortex. Even if you have had a hysterectomy, you still produce some progesterone and some estrogen.

Measuring progesterone levels is the easiest way to determine the time of ovulation, because that's when progesterone levels surge. It is also helpful for determining if a pregnancy is strong enough to carry a baby to term. A low level of progesterone can lead to a miscarriage.

Women concerned about determining whether menopause is close at hand should be tested for progesterone during ovulation. If the score is low or erratic, then menopause is either approaching or has arrived.

Both men and women make progesterone, testosterone and estrogen. Having a balanced progesterone level is the key to regulating estrogen and testosterone. Women generally make more estrogen and men make more testosterone. The solution to any imbalance is usually to address the progesterone level and not the individual estrogen or testosterone levels. Females who do not menstruate and adult males usually have very low scores. In order to fully understand this score, you should review your Official Laboratory Results for further details.

60. Sickle Cell

Sickle cell anemia occurs when red blood cells assume an irregular shape due to a malformation of hemoglobin. It is often confused with a disease called Hemoglobin S Beta Thalassemia.

People who inherit the sickle cell gene from only one parent are usually immune to malaria (a disease prevalent in Africa), and are less likely to have clotting problems. However, if both parents have the sickle cell gene, blood clotting can be a serious problem and premature death may be more likely. It is believed that this cell malformation may have been the effect of a genetic change to protect Africans from malaria.

The sickle-shaped red blood cells have more difficulty moving through blood vessels. Lack of proper hemoglobin and the resulting reduced oxygen-carrying capacity, as well as increased sluggishness of red blood cell movement, causes many sickle cell sufferers to be exhausted. A "sickle cell crisis" occurs when bundles of these irregular cells cause a bottleneck type of blockage in various blood vessels. These serious blockages can be debilitating, very painful and lead to organ damage.

The sickle cell test is very specific in its methodology for establishing accurate results. This test is essential for those of African descent.

Eicosapentaenoic (EPA) acid is an oil found in fish, and available in supplemental form. EPA can make the sickle cells flow more freely, thereby lowering the frequency of blood-cell blockages.

A negative score means you do not have sickle cell anemia. This is the desired result. A positive value indicates the presence of sickle cells.

61. Serum Homocysteine

Homocysteine is an amino acid formed by the body as a byproduct of methionine metabolism. (Methionine is an essential amino acid protein.) Your body needs homocysteine, but it should be broken down after it has done its job. A lack of the enzymes required to break it down and/or a lack of certain B vitamins may allow high levels of homocysteine to accumulate in your bloodstream. (B-vitamin deficiency can be caused by insufficient intake and stress.) Homocysteine begins to attack blood vessel walls, which causes platelets to stick together and promotes free radical damage to the inside of arteries.

Researchers conclude that homocysteine is up to forty times more predictive for assessing cardiovascular disease risk than cholesterol. A score of 15 is the highest acceptable score. From 5 to 15 is the average Lab Reference Range but preferred scores are below 5. Vitamin B_6, B_{12} and folic acid assist the breakdown of homocysteine and help to keep the level as low as possible.

A score higher than 15 is called hyperhomocysteinemia. A less than optimum score is usually the result of having an improper intake of B complex vitamins (including vitamin B_6, EPA fish oil and lycoprene). Additional testing would be necessary to identify the amount needed for these nutrients.

62. Ferritin

Ferritin refers to iron stored in tissues such as the liver, spleen and bone marrow. Ferritin levels are lower when there is an iron deficiency in the cells, and higher when there is an overload in the cells. Therefore, ferritin levels are useful in evaluating the body's total storage of iron.

A score that is less than 10 indicates anemia, or lack of iron inside the cells. It is important to note that one may have enough iron in the blood but cells that are not able to utilize it. One cause may be an excess of iron in household plumbing pipes or well water filled with an unusable form of iron.

Women who have heavy and more frequent menstrual cycles are sometimes anemic and can have lower ferritin levels. Pregnant women have lower than normal levels because more iron is needed by the developing fetus. Blood may also be lost during delivery which depletes iron. Ferritin levels are higher in men and increase in women after menopause. Levels may be higher due to alcoholism, hyperthyroidism and inflammatory diseases like hepatitis.

Rheumatoid arthritis is associated with a low iron level in the blood. A decrease in ferritin along with an increase in your c-reactive protein score (which is explained on the next page) can alert you to an impending rheumatoid arthritis attack.

A score above the Lab Reference Range indicates:
- Excessive iron inside cells
- Severe inflammation, as with arthritis
- Iron overload with damage to the liver
- Malignancy such as leukemia and lymphoma *(note*

other test scores before jumping to diagnostic conclusions; consult your doctor)

A score below the Lab Reference Range indicates:
- Anemia or low iron inside cells
- A low hemoglobin score as well
- Stress (iron can be destroyed by stress)

63. hs-CRP (C-Reactive Protein)

The highly sensitive C-Reactive Protein test indicates the presence of acute injury, inflammation or infection. Since bacterial infection scores are usually higher than viral infection scores, the hs-CRP test is often used to distinguish between the two when infection is present. Increased inflammation, inadequate circulation and poor cellular oxygenation can affect your hs-CRP score. A hs-CRP elevated *above the lab reference range* may indicate Crohn's disease, myocardial infarction (heart attack), post-operative surgery infections, herpes, appendicitis, leukemia, fibromyalgia and any other disease involving infection and inflammation (even the common cold and flu). To achieve the lowest possible score, which is the goal, maintain a strong immune system, keep protein intake at an optimum range and balance arachidonic acid. Learn more about arachidonic acid as described in greater detail under the Omega 3 Profile+ test.

A second hs-CRP score, called the CV Risk score, is often generated when the hs-CRP is performed with lipid profile or full cholesterol series including triglycerides. The reason for combining the results of these tests is that you are more likely to have a future heart attack with less than optimum cholesterol and triglyceride scores.

A score above the lab reference range indicates:
- An impending arthritis attack
- A risk of heart attack
- An impending inflammatory disease attack
- A strong need to test Omega 3 Profile+

64. Isoenzymes

Isoenzyme is a test that is usually ordered when a high alkaline phosphatase level has been identified. It is done to determine whether an initial Alkaline Phosphatase test result was high because of a problem with the bones or skeletal system, the liver, the pancreas, intestinal system or some combination of these.

The following is only a guide to help you understand the isoenzyme results. This test is complicated and not easy to interpret. It should be analyzed by a physician.

A score above the Lab Reference Range can indicate:
- A broken bone
- Osteoblastic tumor (bone tumor)
- Paget's disease (chronic inflammation of bones with thickening and distortion)
- Cancer of the bones, liver, pancreas or intestines

Again we would like to re-emphasize that this test is only meaningful if an Alkaline Phosphatase test result is above the lab normal reference range.

65. Fasting Insulin

Before the body can use any kind of food it must be broken down into glucose. Your pancreas secretes insulin as needed to lower blood sugar levels so that the nutrients can be used efficiently. The amount of insulin sent into the body is just enough to break down the food being eaten when you have a balanced system. When your insulin production is erratic, the metabolism is also erratic. This can alter mood and/or weight management.

Carbohydrates in your diet usually stimulate insulin secretion. Insulin is actually a storage hormone that drives the carbohydrates, protein and fats, all of which must be broken down into glucose, into the cells for either immediate use or long-term storage. High insulin levels prevent the release of stored body fat from the adipose tissue (fat). YFH has found that stress, as well as the over-consumption of high carbohydrate and high glycemic foods, can cause irregular production of insulin. This creates a situation, called insulin resistance, in your body where excessive amounts of insulin are needed to do the work that should be accomplished by far less. *Insulin can cause problems with inflammation, and people with a score over 10 MCIU/ML have a greater possibility of developing heart disease than do those with elevated LDL cholesterol levels.* The fasting insulin test measures the amount of insulin present in your blood even though you are fasting. Controlling your diet and managing your stress are the keys to regular insulin production and reaching the goal of a 5.0 score.

66. Hemoglobin A-1-c Fractionation

The Hemoglobin A-1-c Fractionation takes glucose testing one step further than the traditional fasting glucose test. Although usually ordered for diabetics, this test can be valuable even for non-diabetics because it provides an *average glucose level* over the previous 6 weeks prior to testing. It is possible to have an excellent glucose score one day and an imperfect score the next so the Hemoglobin A-1-c Fractionation is more accurate than a traditional fasting glucose test ordered independently. The life cycle of a red blood cell is 100-120 days. During this lifetime, an irreversible glucose-protein bond continues through the life of an erythrocyte or red blood cell. This test, which is done on a red blood cell, measures the level of glucose present throughout the lifespan of the red blood cell. This average level helps the diabetic or hypoglycemic to assess if the program for dietary balance they are following is actually working. Achieving a score of 4.5 within the range of 3.0 to 6.0 is optimum for most people on this test.

67. VAP

This exciting new expanded genetic cholesterol test is the most powerful available today. This is one of the critical tests YFH believes will make heart disease a thing of the past, especially if used in combination with the Omega 3 Profile+ AA/EPA ratio. VAP differs from routinely run cholesterol tests in critical ways. The expanded VAP test provides all the scores the basic test supplies, but is more detailed and indicates whether the problem is genetic, poor diet, exercise-related, supplement deficiency, ineffective cholesterol medication or a combination of the these. *Some medications given with the best intentions sometimes enhance the formulation of the worst lipoproteins.* Conventional cholesterol testing includes the total cholesterol level, HDL (high-density lipoprotein) "good", LDL (low-density lipoprotein) "bad", and VLDL (very low-density lipoprotein) "worst". With the latest technology and advanced equipment done with the VAP, these 3 categories can no longer be considered as all good or bad. There are fluffy/protective and dense/non-protective divisions within all 3 categories! The VAP breaks down each of the 3 cholesterol types into quantities present of each type.

The goal is:
- To have mostly fluffy/protective HDLs
- As few LDLs and VLDLs as possible with most of them being the fluffy/protective type
- In all categories you want as few dense/non-protective as possible

The VAP goes even further by providing patterns A, AB and B. These refer to your genetic predisposition to a life with cholesterol problems. The belief was that genetic scores could not be changed, **not true**. The correct amount of EPA fish oil, diet, exercise and supplementation (in some cases, medication) can change your predisposition to cardiovascular disease even if it is "in the genes." Remember, total cholesterol may be low, but still be deadly. This explains why healthy people drop dead of a heart attack. Dying of heart disease is no longer *your* fate just because it was your parents'. The earlier you receive information, the sooner you can correct the hand nature dealt you.

68. Omega 3 Profile + (Includes Serum AA/EPA Ratio and Omega 3 Score)

At the time of this printing, this test is the only one of its kind in the world. It is already proving invaluable for improving Cardiovascular Disease, Diabetes, ADD, Multiple Sclerosis, Fibromyalgia, Chronic Fatigue syndrome, fertility issues, cognitive impairment, Alzheimers, depression, and thyroid dysfunction.

This Omega 3 Profile+ test consists of 35 serum plasma essential fatty acids (EFA's). It has two unique component parts. The first part, called the AA/EPA ratio, is an inflammation biomarker. The other, called the Omega 3 Score, is a cardiovascular risk assessment. Results of ten years of research are documented in the reference section in Part IV and in "Heart Disease—No More!" in Part I. Having the proper score can make you 70% less likely to die of a heart attack.

Essential fatty acids are needed by your body to function properly and to protect itself against diseases. Your body does not produce these fatty acids. They must be present in the correct quantities or inflammation and disease can follow. The other five essential fatty acid scores identified by this test are: EPA (Eicosapentaenoic Acid), DHA (Docosahexaenoic Acid), ALA (Flax), AA (Arachidonic Acid), and GLA (Gamma Linoleic Acid).

EPA and DHA are omega 3 long chain fatty acids that are found mainly in salmon, mackerel, herring, sardines and tuna fish oil. They are critical for optimum cardiovascular and brain function.

ALA is a short chain fatty acid found primarily in flaxseed and flaxseed oil. Some of the short chain fatty acids are converted into the needed long chain fatty acids in our bodies but for many people at a very low rate. You may need both long chain and short chain fatty acids to have a balanced system. The test provides the data to know.

Arachidonic acid, an essential fatty acid, is needed by the body but not in excess. When too much is produced, inflammation occurs in your system. Research has shown that this inflammation is a direct cardiovascular risk. It is most often silent. That is, you cannot feel it. There are no symptoms that you have inflammation until the score is very high. Once the level is high enough, symptoms will appear. By testing before symptoms appear, one can find disease early and lower AA levels to prevent the pain that accompanies higher levels. For more information on AA, please read Marcia Yager's story in the case study section and visit www.ZoneLabs.com.

GLA is an omega 6 essential fatty acid. A strong immune system depends on this level remaining adequate in the blood. Most of the people we test have scores less than 0.05 and many have zero scores. It is possible to have too much of this particular omega 6, but so far we have never found anyone with an elevated score.

Please note that there are other EFA tests, but they do not perform the analysis on plasma. Those tests are done on a whole red blood cell, which does not produce an accurate score for tracking a trend. The Omega 3 Profile+ test is quite unique and time consuming to do, but the benefit is worth the cost and the time. Doing this test to get a baseline for these EFA's is one of the most important tests one can do.

Blood Tests to Track for

Specific Illnesses and Symptoms

(Early Detection & Prevention)

After more than two decades of clinical work, YFH has developed an extensive range of data on blood test results that can correlate to specific problems and illnesses. We list illness and symptom categories here, along with their corresponding blood tests that have responded to nutritional balancing. A list of the names of these tests is provided on the next page.

These are the areas that you'll want to focus on first, if you have a specific problem, or are trying to prevent an illness for which you may have a hereditary risk factor. All of the tests listed are important for correcting that symptom or problem but the special focus tests are particularly critical.

It's important to note that much of what we list here is based on our own extensive research. To achieve the best results, you'll need to balance your blood according to a much more specific standard than that of most lab "normal" reference ranges. Nutritional needs, regardless of blood type, are unique to each individual. The accurate interpretation of comprehensive blood tests can tell us the specific nutritional needs of each person and which foods need to be added or deleted from the basic group of foods that are suggested for the blood type.

Test Categories and Their Specific Measures

1. **Electrolytes**
   Sodium
   Potassium
   Chloride
   Bicarbonate
   Glucose

2. **Minerals**
   Phosphorus
   Calcium
   Magnesium*
   Zinc*
   Iron

3. **Bones**
   Alkaline
   Phosphatase

4. **Kidneys**
   BUN
   Creatinine
   BUN/Creatinine
      Ratio
   Uric Acid

5. **Protein**
   Total Protein
   Albumin
   Globulin
   Albumin/Globulin
      Ratio

6. **Liver/Heart**
   GGTP
   SGOT
   SGPT
   LDH
   Bilirubin Total &
      Direct

7. **Complete Blood Count**
   WBC
   RBC
   HGB
   HCT
   Platelets
   MCV
   MCH
   MCHC
   RDW
   Manual RBC
      Morphology

8. **Manual RBC Morphology***
   Anisocytosis
   Microcytosis
   Macrocytosis
   Hypochromasia
   Polychromasia
   Poikilocytosis
   Ovalocytosis
   Elliptocytosis
   Target Cells

9. **Lipid Profile**
   Total Cholesterol
   HDL
   Cholesterol/HDL
      Ratio
   LDL
   Triglycerides
   TG/HDL

10. **WBC Details/ Manual Differential***
    Neutrophils
    Eosinophils
    Lymphocytes
    Monocytes
    Basophils
    Bands
    Atypical
    Lymphocytes

11. **Thyroid Panel II & Free T4**
    T3 Uptake
    T4
    FT7 Index
    Free T4
    TSH

12. **Cancer Tests**
    PSA
    PSAII
    CA125
    CEA
    CA-15-3
    CA-19-9

13. **Special Tests**
    Progesterone
    Sickle Cell
    Serum
       Homocysteine
    Ferritin
    Hs-CRP C-Reactive
       Protein
    Fasting Insulin
    A-1-C Hemoglobin
    VAP
    Omega 3 Profile+

* Tests are more expensive and therefore rarely ordered in most comprehensive panels. It is these tests that provide you extra value. Categories 1 thru 10 are included in a Basic HealthPrint. Categories 11 thru 13 are available at an additional cost.

Symptoms, Illnesses & Diseases Reference List

(*INDICATES TESTS NOT INCLUDED IN A BASIC HEALTHPRINT)

Acne/Psoriasis
Special Focus: Omega 3 Profile +, Progesterone*, Zinc*

Kidneys	Lipid Profile	Liver
Minerals	Protein	WBC Details/Manual Differential

Allergies
Special Focus: Eosinophils, Omega 3 Profile +, Zinc*

Liver	Minerals
Protein	WBC Details/Manual Differential

Arthritis
Special Focus: Alkaline Phosphatase, C-Reactive Protein (hs-CRP), Ferritin*, Magnesium, Omega 3Profile +*, Zinc*

CBC	Manual RBC/	Protein
Electrolytes	Morphology	Custom Thyroid
Free T4*	Minerals	Panel II*
Liver	Progesterone*	WBC Details/ Manual Differential

Cancer
Special Focus: Atypical Lymphocytes, Bands, CA-125 (Women), CA-15-3*, CA-19-9*, CBC, CEA*,C-Reactive Protein*, Ferritin*, Omega 3 Profile +*, PSAII (Men)*, Zinc*

Alkaline Phosphatase	Manual RBC/	Protein
Electrolytes	Morphology	WBC Details/Manual
Liver	Minerals	Differential

Diabetes/Hypoglycemia
Special Focus: A-1-c Hemoglobin, CA-19-9*,Fasting Insulin*, Homocysteine*, Omega 3 Profile+*, Protein, Triglycerides, Zinc, VAP**

CBC	Electrolytes	Lipid Profile
C-Reactive Protein*	Kidneys	Minerals Protein

222

Energy Hyper/Hypo
Special Focus: CBC, CEA*, Ferritin*, Free T4*, Iron, Manual RBC Morphology, Omega 3 Profile+*, Potassium, Sickle Cell (African Descent)*, Custom Thyroid Panel II*, Zinc

Electrolytes	Liver	Protein
Lipid Profile	Minerals	WBC Details/Manual Differential

Fertility Disorders
Special Focus: CA-125 (Women)*, CBC, CEA*, Calcium, Ferritin*, FreeT4*, Glucose, Iron, Magnesium, Manual RBC Morphology, Omega 3 Profile+*, Progesterone*, Protein, Custom Thyroid Panel II*, Zinc

Electrolytes	Liver	WBC Details/Manual
Lipid Profile	Minerals	Differential

Fibromyalgia
Special Focus: CBC, CEA*, Calcium, Ferritin*, Free T4*, Glucose, Magnesium, Omega 3 Profile+*, Potassium, Progesterone*, Custom Thyroid Panel II*, VAP*, WBC Details/Manual Differential, Zinc

Electrolytes	Liver	Protein
Lipid Profile	Minerals	RDW*

Heart Disease/High Cholesterol
Special Focus: Calcium, C-Reactive Protein*, Glucose, Homocysteine*, LDH, Magnesium, Omega 3Profile+*, SGOT, VAP*

Electrolytes	Liver	Minerals
Fasting Insulin*	Protein	Custom Thyroid
Free T4*		Panel II*

Hypertension/Blood Pressure Irregularities
Special Focus: CBC, C-Reactive Protein*, Calcium, Free T4*, Glucose, Homocysteine*, Magnesium, Omega 3 Profile+*, Potassium, Protein, Sodium, Custom Thyroid Panel II*, VAP*

Electrolytes	Lipid Profile	Manual RBC/
Kidneys	Liver	Morphology
Minerals		

Immune System Strength
Special Focus: CA-125 (Women)*, CA-15-3 (Women)*, CA-19-9*, CEA*, C-Reactive Protein*, Omega 3 Profile+*, PSA II (Men)*, WBC Details/Manual Differential, Zinc

CBC	Manual RBC/	Minerals
Ferritin*	Morphology	Protein
Liver		

Migraines
Special Focus: CEA*, Electrolytes, Progesterone*, Manual RBC Morphology, Omega 3 Profile+*, Zinc

Alkaline Phosphatase	Homocysteine*	PSA II (Men)*
CA-125 (Women)*	Lipid Profile	C-Reactive Protein*
CBC	Liver	Custom Thyroid
Ferritin*	Minerals	Panel II*
Free T4*	Protein	WBC Details/Manual Differential

Osteoporosis
Special Focus: Alkaline Phosphatase, CEA*, Calcium, Free T4*, Magnesium, Omega 3 Profile+*, Progesterone*, Custom Thyroid Panel II*, Zinc

Minerals	Protein

PMS/Menopause
Special Focus: CA-125 (Women)*, CA-15-3 (Women)*, CEA*, FreeT4*, Glucose, Omega 3 Profile+*, Potassium, Progesterone*, Magnesium, Custom Thyroid Panel II*, Zinc

Electrolytes	Ferritin*	Minerals
Protein		

Sleep Problems
Special Focus: Calcium, Free T4*, Magnesium, Omega 3 Profile+*, Progesterone*, Custom Thyroid Panel II*, Zinc

CBC	Manual RBC/	Minerals
Electrolytes	Morphology	Protein

Weight Loss/Gain
Special Focus: CA-125 (Women)*, Calcium, CEA*, Free T4*, Omega 3 Profile+*, Potassium, Progesterone*, Sodium, Custom Thyroid Panel II*, Zinc

CBC	Electrolytes	Kidneys
Protein		

Test Suggestions

These test groups are valuable tools to protect your health. Monitoring these results can alert you to possible potential disease long before symptoms develop. Treatment is most successful when disease is detected in the earliest stages.

Women – Basic HealthPrint plus:

Omega 3 Profile +*	CA-19-9*	C-Reactive Protein*
CA-125*	CEA*	Progesterone*
CA-15-3*	Ferritin*	VAP*
Custom Thyroid Panel II*	Free T4*	Homocysteine*

Men – Basic HealthPrint plus:

Omega 3 Profile+*	Progesterone*	C-Reactive Protein*
CA-19-9+	Ferritin*	PSA II*
CEA*	Homocysteine*	VAP*
Free T4*	Custom Thyroid Panel II*	

References and Suggested Reading

Alford, Susan. Personal Interview. May 16, 2000.

Atkins, Robert C. *Dr. Atkins' Diet Revolution.* New York: Bantam, 1973.

Atkins, Robert C. *Dr. Atkins' New Diet Revolution.* New York: Avon, 1992.

Atkins, Robert C. *Dr. Atkins' New Carbohydrate Gram Counter.* New York: M. Evans and Company, 1996.

"American Journal of Clinical Nutrition", Based on Lemaitre *et al.*, 77:319, 2003

"American Journal of Epidemiology", Determined from Simon *et al.*, 42:469, 1995

Balch, Phyllis A.-CNC and James F. Balch MD *Prescription for Nutrition Healing*, 3rd Edition, Avery-Putnam, Inc., 2000

Bass, Stanley S. "Improving Your Diet May Cause You To Feel Sick." http://www.angelfire.com/ny2/bass/symptoms.html 1984.

Bethea, Morrison C. "Break the Sugar Habit, Lose Weight...Feel Great." Interview with *Bottom Line* 15 Oct 1998.

Chase, Marilyn. "Blood Work Reveals Just How Healthy Or Sick You Are." *Wall Street Journal,* 22 Jan 1996, Health Journal.

Clayman, Charles B. The American Medical Association: *Home Medical Encyclopedia.* 2 vols. New York: Random House, 1989.

D'Adamo, Peter, and Catherine Whitney. *Eat Right For Your Type.* New York: Putnam, 1996.

Fackelmann, Kathleen. "Stress, Unhealthy Habits Costing USA." *USA Today,* 3 Oct 2000.

Frohse, Franz, Max Bröedel, Leon Schlossberg. 6th ed. *Atlas of Human Anatomy.* New York: Barnes & Noble Inc., 1961.

Gaby, Alan R., and Jonathan V. Wright. *Nutritional Therapy In Medical Practice*. Kent: Wright/Gaby Seminars, 1996.

Gittleman, Ann Louise. *The Fat Flush Plan*. New York: McGraw-Hill Professional Publishing, 2001.

Gittleman, Ann Louise. *Before The Change*. San Francisco: Harper San Francisco, 1999.

Gittleman, Ann Louise. *Eat Fat, Lose Weight*. New York: McGraw Hill, 2001.

Goldberg, Burton and Editors of Alternative Medicine. *Weight Loss: An Alternative Medicine Definitive Guide*. Payallup: Future Medicine Publishing Inc., 2000.

Griffith, H. Winter. *Complete Guide To Symptoms, Illness & Surgery*. New York: The Putnam Publishing Group, 1989.

Jacobs, David S., et al. *Laboratory Test Handbook: C*O*N*C*I*S*E with Disease Index*. Hudson: Lexi-Comp, 1996.

Kamen, Betty. *She's Gotta Have It!* Novato: Nutrition Encounter, 2001.

Kamen, Betty. *Hormone Replacement Therapy: Yes or No?* Novato: Nutrition Encounter, 1996.

Kamen, Betty. *New Facts About Fiber.* Novato: Nutrition Encounter, 1991.

Kimber, Diane Clifford, et al. *Anatomy and Physiology.* 14th ed. New York: The MacMillan Company, 1962.

Kirschman, John D. *Nutrition Almanac.* 1st ed. New York: McGraw-Hill Book Company, 1975.

Kliman, Bernard, Raymond Vermette and Ernest Kolowrat. *What You Should Know About Medical Lab Tests.* New York: Thomas Y. Crowell, 1979.

Lininger, Schuyler W., et al. *A-Z Guide To Drug-Herb-Vitamin Interactions.* Roseville: Prima Publishing, 1999.

Lininger, Schuyler W., et al. *The Natural Pharmacy.* Roseville: Prima Publishing, 1999.

Long, Howard C. *An Approach to Total Wellness.* American Physical Fitness Research Institute.

McDonald, Arline, Annette Natow and Jo-Ann Heslin. *Complete Book of Vitamins & Minerals.* Lincolnwood: Publications International, Ltd., 1993.

Mikkelson, Barbara. *Readings Railroaded* "CA-125" Last updated: 14 April 2000.

Miller, Bruce B. *Why Food Supplements.* Fort Worth: Bruce Miller Enterprises, Inc., 1982.

Miller, Bruce B. *Your Water...Is It Safe To Drink?* 2nd ed. Fort Worth: Bruce Miller Enterprises, Inc., 1994.

Nano, Stephanie. "U.S.-Italian study finds new data that show heart can repair itself." *The Orlando Sentinel* 3 January 2002, p. A1.

Proudfit, Fairfax T. and Corrine H. Robinson. *Normal and Therapeutic Nutrition.* 12th ed. New York: The MacMillan Company, 1965.

Rasmussen, Oscar. Personal Interview. July 10, 2000.

Robertson, Donald S. "Water, How 8 Glasses a Day Keeps Fat Away." *The Snowbird Diet.*

Schiller, Jack G. *Childhood Illness, A Common Sense Approach.* New York: Stein and Day Publishers, 1972.

Sears, Barry. *The Zone.* New York: HarperCollins Publishers, 1995.

Sears, Barry. *The Omega RX Zone.* New York: HarperCollins Publishers, 2002.

Siegel, Bernie S. Love, *Medicine & Miracles.* New York: Harper & Row Publishers, 1986.

Steward, H. Leighton, et al. *Sugar Busters! Cut Sugar To Trim Fat.* New York: Ballantine, 1998.

Steward, H. Leighton, et al. *Sugar Busters! Shopper's Guide.* New York: Ballantine, 1999.

Taber, Clarence Wilbur. *Taber's Cyclopedic Medical Dictionary.* 10th ed. Philadelphia: F.A. Davis Company, 1965.

Urban Legend. "Primary Peritoneal Cancer." Private e-mail message, (www.urbanlegends.com).

Vickery, Donald M. and James F. Fries. *Take Care of Yourself, The Consumers Guide To Medical Care.* 3rd ed. Reading, Mass: Addison-Wesley Publishing Co., 1986.

Werbach, Melvyn R. *Nutritional Influences on Illness.* 2nd ed. Tarzana: Third Line Press, 1993.

Wheeler, Margaret F. and Wesley A. Volk. *Basic Microbiology.* Philadelphia: J.B. Lippincott Company, 1964.

Winslow, Ron. "Gender study Suggests Heart can Repair Itself." *The Wall Street Journal* 3 January 2002, pp. B1,B3.

World Book: Rush-Presbyterian-St. Luke's Medical Center, Medical Encyclopedia. Chicago: World Book, 1991.

Wright, Karen. "The Clot Thickens." *Discover,* Dec 1999.

Wurtman, Judith. "Power Eating, Foods to Make You More Productive." Interview with *Bottom Line.*

GLOSSARY

AMINO ACIDS - The building blocks of a protein molecule.

ANTIOXIDANTS - A substance capable of protecting other substances from oxidation.

BALANCING YOUR pH - By balancing your pH levels you can find the quantity of carbohydrates your body needs to gain, lose or maintain weight. This balancing also helps to improve your kidney, blood sugar and cholesterol scores.

EDEMA - Retention of fluids within the body, causing swelling.

HEALTHPRINT - A nutritional blood test interpretation system service by YFH.

HEALTH SCORECARD - This is the "How am I doing today?" report which compares your blood test scores to your customized optimum ranges. The suggestion column identifies tests that need to be improved. It provides the test category, test name, lab analysis reference range and optimum suggestions as well as notations of any equipment or range changes from your previous test time.

HEMOGLOBIN - Iron-containing pigment of the red blood cells.

HEMOLYSIS - Destruction of red blood cells.

LABORATORY "NORMAL" REFERENCE RANGE - An inconsistent reference, which compares your blood test results against broad population averages.

OFFICIAL LAB RESULTS - Blood test results from the laboratory, in the laboratory format, to be interpreted by a health care professional.

OPTIMUM RANGE - This is the range that YFH computes to be most optimum for you each time you test. It is based on your age, gender, height, weight and other blood test scores.

PERSONAL NORMAL LEVEL - Repeated testing develops your unique benchmark level for each test.

PERSONAL NORMAL TRACKER - Your history of all blood tests done with YFH. You use this to find your personal normal levels as you change your foods, exercise, stress level, vitamins, minerals and herbs.

INDEX

Progesterone 71, 76, 100, 122, 201
Prostate 130, 131, 194, 195
PSA 193
PSAII 194
PSA, Total 194

R

Ranges, "sick" 119
Rare Disease 117
RBC 86, 100, 103, 114, 116, 171
RDW 178

S

Scott & Bridget-Infertility 99, 100, 101
SGOT 166
SGPT 167
Shannahan, Duke-Autoimmune, Arthritis 115
Shaner, Ginni-Multiple disease 126
Sickle Cell 172, 178, 206
Sodium 141
Stroke 69, 171
Synthroid 106

T

T3 Uptake 186, 200
T4 201
T4, Free 76, 106, 186, 203
T7 202
Target Cells 180

Thyroid 71, 76, 98, 100, 105, 106, 114, 122, 147, 150, 200, 201, 206, 207
Total Cholesterol 67, 75, 180, 214
Total Protein 154
Toxic Shock Syndrome 113
Triglycerides 17, 81, 186
TSH 106, 108, 186, 204

U

Urine 18
Uric Acid 159

V

VAP 71, 73, 75, 76, 122, 182, 184, 213

W

WBC 76, 169
Weight 951
Weston, Joyce-Cancer 129
Wolfe, Lena-Rare Disease 118

Z

Zinc 70, 90, 100, 101, 103, 114, 116, 119, 152

Notes

Notes

About the Author

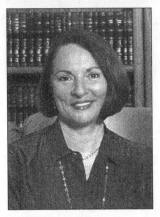

Ellie Cullen has been a licensed Registered Nurse for more than thirty years. She trained at Johns Hopkins, and has over twenty-five years of extensive clinical nursing, nutrition and lifestyle consulting experience. She has personally overcome arthritis and low blood sugar using her YFH system. Ellie has lectured for doctors and health organizations for the last twenty-four years and has clients all over the world.

"I hope every person who reads this book will take the time to share it with not only those friends and family members who are ill, but those who wish to avoid illness. The benefit is even greater to those who are healthy and who wish to remain healthy. My special plea is to test children as well as the elderly. Many believe that children are too young to need preventive testing and that our senior citizens are too old to benefit from it. It is never too early or too late to improve your health."

Ellie Cullen